Advances in Preventing and Treating Violence and Aggression

Series Editor

Peter Sturmey
Queens College and The Graduate Center
City University of New York
Flushing, USA

The series publishes books focused and developed across three domains. The first is understanding and explaining violence and aggression. Books in this domain address such subject matter as genetics, physiology, neurobiology, cultural evolution, biobehavioral, learning, cognitive, psychoanalytic, sociological and other explanations of violence. The second domain focuses on prevention and treatment for individuals and couples. Examples of books in this domain include cognitive behavioral, behavioral, counseling, psychopharmacological, psychosocial, couples, and family therapy approaches. They also explore extant treatment packages for individually focused treatments (e.g., mindfulness, cognitive analytic therapies). Within this domain, books focus on meeting the information needs of clinicians and professionals who work in youth facilities, emergency rooms, special education, criminal justice, and therapy settings. Finally, books in the third domain address prevention and treatment for groups and society, including topical focus on early intervention programs, school violence prevention programs, policing strategies, juvenile facility reform as well as socio-legal and ethical issues. Books in this series serve as must-have resources for researchers, academics, and upper-level undergraduate and graduate students in clinical child and school psychology, public health, criminology/criminal justice, developmental psychology, psychotherapy/counseling, psychiatry, social work, educational policy and politics, health psychology, nursing, and behavioral therapy/rehabilitation.

Tony Ward • Gwenda M. Willis
David S. Prescott • Stijn Vandevelde
Mary Barnao • Wouter Wanzeele

The Good Lives Model of Correctional Rehabilitation

Integrating Theory, Research, and Practice

Springer

Tony Ward
School of Psychology
Victoria University of Wellington
Wellington, New Zealand

David S. Prescott
Safer Society Foundation
Middlebury, VT, USA

Mary Barnao
Central City Psychology
Wellington, New Zealand

Gwenda M. Willis
School of Psychology
University of Auckland
Auckland, New Zealand

Stijn Vandevelde
Department of Special Needs Education
Ghent University
Ghent, Belgium

Wouter Wanzeele
Forensisch Ambulant Begeleidingsteam
CAW Oost-Vlaanderen
Ghent, Belgium

ISSN 2946-4757 ISSN 2946-4765 (electronic)
Advances in Preventing and Treating Violence and Aggression
ISBN 978-3-031-95558-7 ISBN 978-3-031-95559-4 (eBook)
https://doi.org/10.1007/978-3-031-95559-4

This Springer imprint is published by the registered company Springer Nature Switzerland AG
The registered company address is: Gewerbestrasse 11, 6330 Cham, Switzerland

To William (Bill) Marshall

Bill, five of us had the good fortune to spend time with you during our careers. You encouraged, inspired, taught, mentored, challenged, and supported us at different times. As you did with so many other emerging researchers and clinicians. To say we all learned from you is an understatement. Your stellar intellect, creativity, and encyclopedic knowledge of the sexual offending field is obvious to everyone who has opened one of your books or read one of your papers. And certainly, we all benefited from your gifts. What may not be as apparent to those who did not know you personally was your great sense of humor, deep compassion and belief in the capacity of the clients you worked with to change. Somehow you always managed to find a way to connect with them at a human level. It has been such a privilege to know you, Bill. The field is diminished by your loss but enriched by your work. We will miss you.

Preface

Workshop participants often ask about the origins of the Good Lives Model (GLM), namely, where did the idea come from to reorient rehabilitation to incorporate strengths as well as address risk? The story is an interesting one and underlines the crucial role that theory plays in therapy and practice more generally. In 2002 Tony Ward was editing Claire Stewart's PhD thesis on needs assessment in the area of intellectual disability. Her thesis included an excellent review of human needs theory and its implications for identifying intervention needs for individuals with an intellectual disability. At this time, Tony was director of the University of Melbourne's forensic psychology program and upon reading Claire's thesis became increasingly interested in the relationship between human needs and criminogenic needs. As part of this project, he read widely on the topics of wellbeing, human rights, happiness, human needs, quality of life, motivation, therapeutic processes, developmental science, philosophy of science, and moral philosophy. Armed with this literature, Tony focused his attention on the assumptions underlying the dominant model of correctional rehabilitation at the time, the risk-need-responsivity model (RNR; Bonta & Andrews, 2017) and become alarmed. In his view, the criminal justice field had become overly preoccupied with risk prediction and management and overlooked a rather simple fact: individuals who have engaged in criminal behavior have the same needs and aspirations of law-abiding citizens. Essentially, in many respects they are people like us. Furthermore, in his view, the RNR model contained several significant conceptual problems that had been surprisingly overlooked. Tony was interested in this omission both as a researcher and clinician, as in his experience poor theory often results in ineffective practice. He wrote a series of early papers arguing for the advantages of developing strength-based approaches in the criminal justice area, suggesting that the personal priorities of people who had committed offences should be explicitly factored into their intervention plans.

The origin of the GLM started with a simple question but has since developed into a comprehensive model of rehabilitation for individuals of all ages who have committed offenses. The first researcher to join the core team was Mayumi Purvis, followed by Gwenda Willis, Pamela Yates, David Prescott, Mary Barnao, Stijn Vandevelde, and Wouter Wanzeele, five of whom are coauthors of this book. In addition, there is larger group of researchers and clinicians who have published papers with members of the core team and contributed to the development of assessment and intervention innovations. We thank you!

The intended audience for this book includes qualified health, criminal justice, social welfare and other professionals who have a solid understanding of psychological assessment and therapeutic practice.[1] The GLM is not a plug and play practice framework and does assume that clinicians can establish good working alliances with clients and are able to balance its twin goals of well-being enhancement and risk reduction. Having said that, this book should provide therapists unfamiliar with the GLM all they need to acquire a good working knowledge of its theory, assessment, and practice techniques and apply this knowledge to their work. A final note, clients have every right to ask us "How can I live my life differently, and secure what matters most to me?" Strength-based approaches such as the GLM can answer this question in ways that make our communities safer[2] while helping clients discover meaningful ways to live.

Wellington, New Zealand — Tony Ward
Auckland, New Zealand — Gwenda M. Willis
Middlebury, VT, USA — David S. Prescott
Ghent, Belgium — Stijn Vandevelde
Wellington, New Zealand — Mary Barnao
Ghent, Belgium — Wouter Wanzeele

References

Bonta, J., & Andrews, D. A. (2017). *The psychology of criminal conduct* (6th ed.). New York, NY: Routledge.

[1] The client group focused on in this book is adults rather than youth. However, where practice with youth departs significantly from that with adults, we comment on this in the relevant sections of the book. A stand-alone volume for working with youth using the GLM is currently being planned.

[2] The book should be read according to the chapter order. The two initial theory chapters are essential reading as they provide the theoretical context for the rest of the book.

Acknowledgement

We would like to thank Louise Lloyd Prescott for her excellent editorial work on this book. Louise painstakingly read every sentence in every chapter and for that we are eternally grateful. She smoothed out the numerous "reading bumps", asked sharp and revealing questions, and pushed us to express ourselves as clearly as possible. You are a star Louise, thank you!

Competing Interests The authors have no competing interests to declare that are relevant to the content of this manuscript.

Ethics Approval The authors declare that this manuscript does not include primary research with human participants.

The authors declare that this manuscript does not include primary studies involving animals.

Contents

List of Figures

List of Tables

Chapter 1
Good Lives Model of Rehabilitation

1.1 Introduction

The work of behavioral change with the most difficult and reviled individuals in our community often seems like an insurmountable undertaking. Practitioners rely heavily on best practice models and research to guide their practice and reinforce treatment programs. Over the past few decades, there has been a growing and understandable emphasis on *managing risk* of reoffending. While risk management approaches have achieved positive results within the treatment context, these results are still modest (Bonta & Andrews, 2017; Fazel et al., 2024).

A remarkable feature of human beings is their ability to plan and modify aspects of themselves and their environments in order to increase their potential for achieving valued outcomes and avoiding harmful ones (Gallagher, 2023; Tomasello, 2022). For example, people will lose weight to look and feel better, cut alcohol consumption to lower blood pressure and repair damaged relationships, or learn to resolve personal conflicts in ways that do not involve violence. In ideal circumstances, people's living environments would contain the societal, cultural, biological, and physical resources they need to succeed in implementing plans for living "good" lives. However, making the best use of psychological and social resources means individuals need to live meaningful, productive lives, for which they require specific sets of skills and knowledge. To use an analogy, there is little point in being surrounded by precious minerals, and plentiful food sources if you lack the tools necessary to "extract" them in useable forms. One way of identifying the internal and external capacities necessary for individuals to live well in their day-to-day environments, is to call them *strengths*.

From the viewpoint of strength-based rehabilitation models such as the Good Lives Model (GLM; Ward & Maruna, 2007), the fundamental purpose of correctional rehabilitation is to help people develop their capacities to be intimate with another person, to manage emotions, and to coordinate their goals effectively and

T. Ward et al., *The Good Lives Model of Correctional Rehabilitation*,
Advances in Preventing and Treating Violence and Aggression,
https://doi.org/10.1007/978-3-031-95559-4_1

adjust them depending on the challenges of the world. In essence, they must learn how to function within the world in an independent and intelligent way. Strength-based rehabilitation initiatives center on agency (i.e., ability to form and implement plans—see below) while accepting that effective and adaptive actions depend on the availability of opportunities and social supports. People can only live well if the outside world is in sync with their desires and associated values.

This chapter presents an overview of the key theoretical ideas constituting the GLM. First, the concept of science-informed practice is reviewed, and its relevance for strength-based practice approaches to correctional rehabilitation is examined. This conceptual framework places the GLM within the wider context of evidence-based practice. Second is a discussion of the black-box method of constructing explanatory theories and arriving at targets of explanations of offending (Ward & Durrant, 2021). The primary advantage of this conceptual model is that it provides a way of linking offense-related problems with well-being considerations, typically a challenging task (Ward & Durrant, 2022). Correctional rehabilitation programs should aim to help people get what matters most to them at the same time as it increases the safety of the community. Third comes an introduction of the concept of practice frameworks, a type of theory that links core values, knowledge assumptions, and practice implications that follow on from these assumptions. In order to use the GLM effectively in practice, therapists need to understand what type of model it is and not to confuse it with treatment or explanatory models. In fact, it is a little bit of both. Finally, the bulk of the chapter describes the three interwoven levels of the GLM: core values, knowledge-related assumptions, and practice guidelines. The ideas presented in this first chapter constitute the skeleton of the GLM, while subsequent chapters expand on the assessment, intervention, and policy implications of these basic commitments. Without a conceptual map to guide practitioners and clients, it is easy to get lost.

1.2 General Theoretical Frameworks

1.2.1 Science-Informed Practice Model

Clinical work has a long tradition of empirically driven practice, in which therapists are encouraged to base their interventions on the best available research evidence and to think critically during the assessment, case formulation, and treatment phases of practice. Training programs typically set out to produce individuals who combine the skills of researchers and therapists within a single professional role (Haynes et al., 1999; Shapiro, 1979). According to the scientist-practitioner model, the aim of clinical inquiry is to produce scientifically grounded explanations of clients' problems, and then select empirically supported interventions specifically designed to address them. The model of evidence-based practice (EBP) is based on this earlier conceptualization of the therapist role and similarly directs clinicians to integrate the best available research evidence to guide therapy assessment and treatment

(Spring & Neville, 2011). However, the EBP model goes beyond the earlier scientist-practitioner model by explicitly incorporating (1) clinical expertise (you need qualified and competent therapists to produce good outcomes); (2) client preferences and values, psychological features, and social and cultural factors into the clinical decision-making process (where clients find meaning is important); alongside (3) empirical evidence supporting the most effective treatment programs underpinned by good theory.

The EBP movement was initially adapted from medicine (Sackett et al., 2000) and has since been adopted across health disciplines as an overarching practice framework (e.g., social work, Drisko & Grady, 2019; nursing, Bucknall & Rycroft-Malone, 2021; forensic psychology, Gannon & Ward, 2014; and clinical psychology, Ward et al., 2022). The American Psychological Association has endorsed the EBP approach and laid down: "Evidence-based practice in psychology (EBPP) is the integration of the best available research with clinical expertise in the context of patient characteristics, culture, and preferences" (APA Presidential Task Force on EBP, 2006, p. 271). In the last 15 years, a transdisciplinary model of EBP has been developed, building on the common elements and unique strengths of each of the social work, medicine, public health, and psychology models (Satterfield et al., 2009).

The original EBM of practice has recently been modified to deal with issues that threatened its theoretical integrity and arguably made it harder to implement in clinical settings (Ward et al., 2022). Changes include the recognition that conceptual analysis; problem formulation; classification; and theory construction, development, and evaluation are all crucial aspects of science and its application to psychological problems. The concept of evidence has been replaced with a less restrictive term "relevant epistemic (knowledge) considerations." This makes it easier to employ different types of argument structures and evidence in research and clinical reasoning. Evidence in this broader sense also encompasses conceptual analysis and theoretical reasoning that can justify a set of hypotheses or claims (Ward et al., 2024a). Evidence is best understood in relation to specific inquiry tasks, and what constitutes the right kind of knowledge depends on the task undertaken and the methods employed to achieve it. Essentially, science is a human practice, and therefore values and goal-directed actions underpin every aspect of it.

The broader conception of the EBP model means that researchers and clinicians need to look beyond the bare research evidence and incorporate clinical expertise along with client core values and biological, psychological, social, and cultural characteristics in treatment recommendations (Gannon & Ward, 2014). Furthermore, clients should be regarded as partners in the change process. Their unique perspectives on their own experiences and lives should be factored into clinical decision-making. The question of what constitutes relevant and reliable evidence and researcher competence depends on the domain and focus of disagreement and so will vary accordingly. Extending this idea to clinical work means that some forms of evidence are best articulated by clients, while practitioners should have constructive knowledge-related dialogues with them to construct valid case formulations and relevant intervention plans. Our aim should be to work alongside clients to arrive at personally meaningful intervention goals and plans, and not just apply treatments to them. This is a significant shift from the typical practice where information provided by clients is treated with suspicion and its significance downgraded. Simply working from a list of dynamic risk factors (DRF) or set of psychometric scales is insufficient to arrive at an understanding of the meaning of offending for individuals convicted of crimes. What is often missing is insight into their priorities, core values, and beliefs. Essentially, we need to remember the client amid all the science.

This enriched EBP is one of the methodological frameworks supporting the GLM with its emphasis on incorporating clients' core values, dignity, and preferences into intervention plans. It also places the GLM squarely within the realm of evidence-based practice where conceptual and normative (values in the form of client priorities) analyses are crucial parts of research and practice. Unlike contemporary risk-oriented approaches to correctional rehabilitation, the GLM recognizes the client as an epistemic (knowledge) agent as well as a partner in the change process. Due to its emphasis on theory and values, it is, therefore, ideally situated within the evidence-based practice model, unlike alternative rehabilitation models, such as the Risk-Need-Responsivity model (RNR; Bonta & Andrews, 2017). The major focus of the RNR is on risk management, and it favors empirical research over the construction and analysis of theories and models. This is out of step with contemporary models of science and knowledge (Haig, 2014; Ward et al., 2024a).

1.2.2 The Black-Box Model and Offense Categories

One challenge facing researchers and clinicians in the criminal justice arena is working out how to connect individuals' well-being needs with their offending behavior in ways that do not minimize the importance of either. There is a danger that focusing primarily on offending pathways will result in the neglect of clients' needs and values, while an exclusive focus on individuals' level of well-being may result in a failure to address genuine risk concerns. The recent paper by Ward and Durrant (2022) on the black-box model of theory construction and target identification represents an attempt to achieve this integration. By doing so, it provides a strong justification for the focus of the GLM on risk *and* well-being concerns.

The black-box construct helps explain the development of scientific knowledge of natural and social phenomena, recognizing that the progress is not always linear (Nathan, 2021). More specifically, it helps researchers to identify and explain phenomena of interest by creating an initial coarse representation (what is called a *black box*) of them, for example, initially labeling complex relational and intimacy needs as "intimacy deficits." As the research process unfolds, researchers "open up" the phenomena black boxes are and provide further, more detailed representations of the clinical phenomena and their causes. An initial coarse description of a problem such as *intimacy deficits* can be translated into more specific and precise problems, such as poor communication skills, fear of rejection by adult partners, impaired perspective-taking skills, and so on. This ultimately results in a nested set of boxes, each depicted in greater detail. It's a bit like Russian dolls where a large doll is opened up to reveal a smaller doll within it, and then this doll is opened up to reveal a yet smaller doll, and so on until you eventually arrive at the smallest doll. In science, however, there is no definitive end to the process of opening black boxes within a research program. The point at which any particular process terminates depends in large part on the interests of researchers and the overall benefits of further investigation; deciding where to start and end is basically a pragmatic decision. A key question is: what stopping point within this specific context will help me to solve the problems I am most interested in?

A pressing question is what concept(s) would be useful for initiating the black boxing dynamic in the forensic and correctional domains: offending behavior or psychological and social problems associated with crime? The problem with starting with offense categories is that they offer little useful information about the structure of underlying problems, and they are also extremely heterogeneous (Ward & Carter, 2019). As it turns out, individuals who have committed the same crime often present very different clinical pictures (Ward & Durrant, 2022). On the other hand, failure to anchor theory and clinical interventions in offense categories, at least to some degree, can result in overlooking crucial moral aspects of crime, potentially minimizing risk concerns. Taking account of this dilemma, it makes sense to begin with a crime-related target, primarily because of its social significance. A good example might include acts of sexual aggression or physical violence directed toward innocent members of the community. One possibility is that an initial black box for explaining crime could be criminal offending, represented in terms of an *agent-action-context* unit (see Fig. 1.1—Ward & Durrant, 2021). The agent-action-context schema is sufficiently general to capture the critical features of offending and places an emphasis on the serious violation of moral and legal norms evident in criminal actions.

Different kinds of offending—such as sexual offending, violent offending, and deliberate fire setting—can be represented using the same basic conceptual unit (agent-action-context) but given a "local" representation in terms of the type of offense or offending behavior. Each of the subcomponents comprising this category can then be examined at different levels from varying theoretical perspectives. For example, *agency* could be categorized according to different types of goals or needs, or even in terms of personality features. While *actions* could be classified in terms of offense pathways or developmental trajectories (Ward & Hudson, 2000). The *contexts* of crime-related actions would include the normative (value) expectations of different roles and situations and hence spell out why a particular action constitutes a crime. From a black-box perspective, the general conceptualization of crime is based on an abstract schema of agent-action-context, while different local conceptual systems flesh this idea out in more concrete and distinct ways.

The black-box model offers considerable clinical flexibility when it comes to the explanation and framing of crime and related psychological and social problems. If the goal is simply to assign individuals to a correctional program, then a relatively simple black-box model based on agents' desires, beliefs, and action plan will

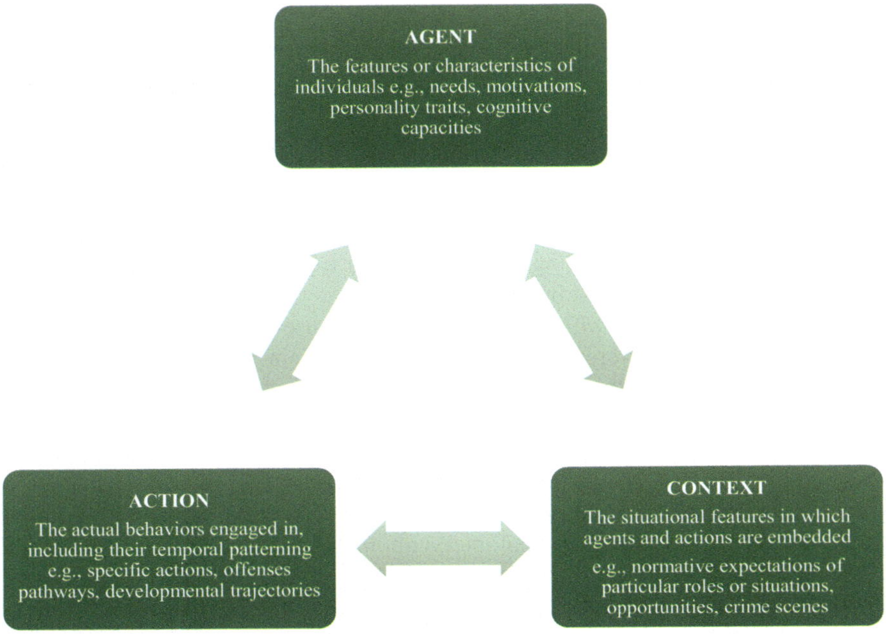

Fig. 1.1 The agent-action-context schema. Reprinted with permission from Ward, T & Durrant, R. (2022). Targets of explanation in forensic and correctional psychology: A black box model. *Aggression and Violent Behavior, 67*, doi.org/10.1016/j.avb.2022.101782

suffice. Questions such as *was the intention to develop a sexual relationship with a child?* and *how did this occur?* will be particularly salient. Thus, framing the relevant explanation targets in terms of general offending behavior is enough. However, for risk prediction purposes, it will be necessary to move down a level to create more detailed black boxes, such as recruiting dynamic risk factors associated with reoffending; e.g., deviant sexual preferences, cognitive distortions, emotional dysregulation, relationship problems (Mann et al., 2010). By way of contrast, explanations intended to guide therapeutic interventions would ideally be based on even more refined black boxes, such as those arising from the deconstruction (breaking down into smaller elements) of risk factors, such as emotional congruence, into finer grained variables like fear of adults, difficulty understanding social situations, seeking a sense of belonging with children, and so on (Ward & Carter, 2019; Ward & Durrant, 2021). The key point is that the type of black box you open and the degree of precision depend on what you are trying to achieve in a specific research or clinical context. There is no single "best interpretative level."

The GLM, with its twin focus on risk reduction and well-being enhancement, is well suited to capitalize on the black-box methodology and the related agent-action-context schema. Assessment will start with the offense and its associated patterns and document what happened, when, and how. Opening the different black boxes of the agent-action-context schema can then provide an explanation of why a person committed an offense (e.g., identifying the relevant primary human goods and motivational systems,-see below) and also specify how non-offending problems are related to the offending behavior. For example, an individual may have committed a sexual offense against children. On analysis it appears that their primary goal was to establish a romantic relationship with a child. The capacity problems associated with their subsequent actions relate to difficulties appreciating other adults' varying perspectives and dealing with their fears of being harmed by them. The context in which offenses occurred are shaped by their goals and capacity impairments and may include virtual pedophilic chatrooms or a world revolving around contact with children. Another individual committing a similar offense, could exhibit completely different sorts of goals and related impairments. Essentially, the black-box model provides a method for deconstructing risk factors (see below) and linking them to offending behaviors. Doing this provides a strong theoretical justification for the GLM's emphasis on risk management and well-being enhancement.

1.2.3 The Practice Framework Model

A practice framework is a new type of theory recently developed by Ward and Durrant (2021), which creates a bridge between treatment theories, normative (value) assumptions, and etiological (explanatory) theories. Ward and Durrant (2021) propose that practice frameworks in the criminal justice domain are composed of three linked sets of ideas or levels (see Fig. 1.2). The three components of the practice framework model are conceptually linked and are hierarchically organized, with each level constraining the one(s) beneath it, a bit like interlocking wheels in a machine. The top level contains normative principles, assumptions, and core values, the second level is concerned with general etiological (causal) and knowledge-related assumptions, and the third includes the broad types of intervention and practice strategies that follow from both the etiological assumptions and core normative commitments. The core values and principles (level 1) spell out what you are trying to achieve, what you need to know to do this (level 2), and how to proceed clinically in light of the values and knowledge assumptions you hold (level 3).

The evaluation of practice frameworks is essentially pragmatic and revolves around the degree to which they provide adequate guidance for intervention. In part, these evaluative criteria are derived from research on the process and outcome of treatment and include factors such as attention to the most effective practitioner style, type of alliance to be formed, within-team and between-team communication and understanding, explicit goals, clear protocols, evidence of efficacy and effectiveness, and stakeholder engagement. The specific evaluation criteria will vary depending on the type of practice framework and the domain in which it is implemented. For example, a treatment-oriented practice framework will need to demonstrate good therapeutic effects while a restorative justice practice framework shows that it can deliver fair outcomes for all the key people involved. In this approach,

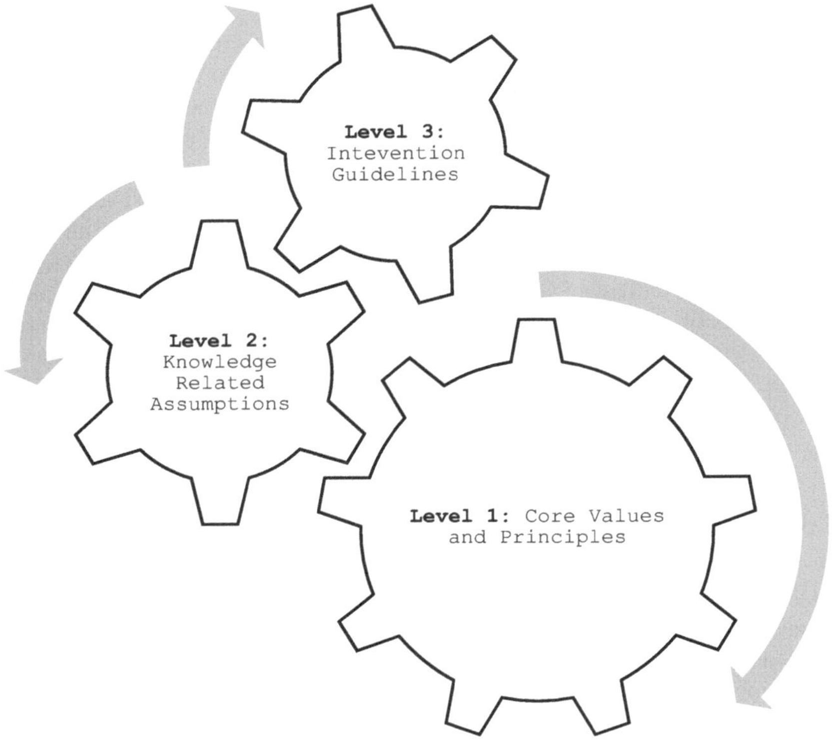

Fig. 1.2 A proposed structure for practice frameworks in correctional psychology. Reprinted with permission from Ward, T. & Durrant, R. (2021). Practice frameworks in correctional psychology: Translating causal theories and normative assumptions into practice. *Aggression and Violent Behavior.* doi.org/10.1016/j.avb.2021.101612

different types of practice frameworks occupy distinct "niches"; essentially, domains of application characterized by their own unique problems. For example, the niche of social reentry and integration requires a practice framework built on desistance ideas (social and personal factors) that reduce the chances of offending when a person is released back into the community (see below), whereas problems like social anxiety or impulsivity require a therapeutically oriented approach.

Practice frameworks in different domains or niches can be used in a coordinated way. Thus, a comprehensive approach to working with individuals who have committed offenses requires the application of complementary but diverse practice frameworks oriented to different problem clusters (niches): (1) response to crime (e.g., restorative justice); (2) dealing with mental health issues (e. g., recovery model); (3) risk prediction and managing risk factors (e.g., Risk-Need-Responsivity Model); (4) enhancing well-being (e.g., Good Lives Model); (5) addressing cultural dislocation (e.g., cultural models); (6) loss of identity (e.g., narrative approaches); and (7) dealing with social reintegration (e.g., desistance models). It is a mistake to see these practice frameworks as always in competition; sometimes they are but often they offer complementary and valuable contributions to crime management and should be used together. The existence of multiple practice frameworks means that practitioners should have a good understanding of the relevant theories in the field they work in and appreciate the need to match an intervention model to the problem. It is a mistake to use a practice model in a domain for which it was not designed, for example, adopting reportative justice as a treatment model when it is better used to address conflicting ethical claims between victims, the community, and individuals who have committed crimes (Ward et al., 2014). They should also be aware of the hybrid nature (i.e., they contain three distinct but interlinked levels) of practice frameworks and the implications of this complexity when it comes to evaluating competing approaches.

1.3 Good Lives Model: Values, Knowledge Assumptions, and Practice Implications[1]

The GLM has a naturalistic view of people and their functioning. It views people as continually evolving beings who are naturally designed to act in the pursuit of a range of biological, psychological, and social goals within certain environments (Arnhart, 1998; Laws & Ward, 2011). These natural desires motivate people to act in ways that they believe will satisfy them. Therefore, any meaningful and effective risk management program needs to consider individuals' associated lifestyles and their environments. To ignore individuals' core motivations is to run the risk of (1) not understanding the reasons why they committed crimes; (2) constructing invalid case formulations and therapy plans; and (3) failing to persuade them to engage fully in intervention programs. Furthermore, dynamic internal risk factors, such as impulsivity or aggressiveness, are only meaningful in terms of the situational, social, and cultural contexts in which they are expressed. Sound intervention should therefore reflect individuals' strengths, values, goals, relevant environments, and contexts and specify precisely what competencies are required to secure valued outcomes in prosocial and personally meaningful ways (Ward, 2010).

The GLM suggests that the best way to prevent harm to the community is through the enhancement of clients' skills and capabilities and actively working toward the achievement of healthy, prosocial goals, rather than simply the avoidance of negative ones. Specifically, the GLM posits that good lives are ways of living that allow an individual to secure *primary human goods* (PHGs; outcomes that are sought for their own sake and have intrinsic value) in personally meaningful ways. According to Ward (2002), all human actions are directly or indirectly linked to the seeking of PHGs, including criminal and antisocial behavior. The goals individuals set for themselves are therefore targeted toward the securing of a human good or goods within the contexts in which they live.

[1] See Appendix E for a glossary of key GLM terms.

1.3.1 Practice Framework Level One: Core Values

The Good Lives Model is grounded in the ethical concepts of human dignity (i.e., Ward, 2011) and universal human rights, and as such it has a strong emphasis on human agency (see below). Essentially, the GLM is concerned with enhancing individuals' ability to formulate and select goals, to construct plans, and to act freely in the implementation of these plans. Although the central aim of the GLM is to build internal and external capacities (i.e., building strengths), it pays equal attention to risk variables and the societal level. It's a responsibility of policymakers within any system to enable people to obtain the resources necessary for individuals to construct and effectively implement their (legal and adaptive) good lives plans. As such, the model advocates for a dual emphasis on risk management and goods promotion. Its core values are reflected in two major normative principles based on these aims.

The GLM has always stressed the importance of viewing individuals as *fellow human beings* (or "fellow travelers") rather than as simply the bearers of risk, and because of this perspective, taking their core needs and concerns seriously. The ethical justification for this humanistic orientation was originally based on human needs and a commitment to developing intervention plans designed to increase clients' levels of well-being (Ward & Stewart, 2003). The subsequent work by Ward and Birgden (2007) strengthened the ethical aspect of the GLM by explicitly linking it to the concepts of human rights and dignity.

The concept of human dignity is an ancient ethical idea that has at its center the claim that every human being has intrinsic worth and is equal in this respect (Waldron, 2009). Initially, it was accepted that individuals' level of dignity varied according to their social status, with serfs considered inferior to nobles or clergy. However, with the event of modern liberal thought in the seventeenth century, a change in meaning occurred. Rather than high value being exclusively associated with individuals of elevated social rank, all human beings were regarded as if they were aristocrats or royalty. Note, however, class differences have not disappeared. Nevertheless, this shift in the meaning of the term dignity in modern times, and its close link with the concept of rights, is well expressed thus:

> Dignity, we are told, was once tied up with rank: the dignity of a king was not the same as the dignity of bishop and neither of them was the same as the dignity of a professor. If our modern conception of human dignity retains any scintilla of its ancient and historical connection with rank—and I think it does: I think it expresses the idea of the high and equal rank of every human person. . . . Dignity is intimately connected with the idea of rights as the ground of rights, and the content of certain rights, and perhaps even the form and structural character of rights (Waldron, 2009, p. 2).

Dignity is a valuable ethical concept, because it is acknowledged as foundational by many individuals whose specific moral theories and codes diverge. Therefore, it is ideally placed to function as an integrative concept for ethical reasoning in these domains (Ward, 2011). Furthermore, in line with other theorists, we propose that there is a close connection between dignity and human rights, but that it is not sufficient to ground practice on its own. What is also needed is the specification of norms that are designed to protect the empowerment and well-being requirements that comprise dignity. The concept of human rights is a moral (and legal) one that can fulfill this role by virtue of its ability to safeguard the provision of the social, economic, environmental, and psychological goods necessary for a dignified human life (Ward & Birgden, 2007). The relationship between values and human rights is well captured by Freeden (1991):

> A human right is a conceptual device, expressed in linguistic form, that assigns priority to certain human or social attributes regarded as essential to the adequate functioning of a human being; that is intended to serve as a protective capsule for those attributes; and that appeal for deliberate action to ensure such protection (p. 7).

Human rights are typically cast in a universal form that applies to all human beings by virtue of their underlying common needs based on the fact of embodiment, environmental conditions, and related interests (Gewirth, 1996). Most theorists assert that human rights are *claim rights* possessed by all human beings that guarantee them access to certain goods such as food, education, and the ability to engage in specific types of actions, such as free speech or freedom of movement (Orend, 2002). These rights can be positive, in that someone has an obligation to supply the goods in question, or negative, whereby there is an obligation not to interfere with someone's activities. Those who enjoy human rights have obligations to others to allow access to specific sets of goods and, in turn, have entitlements to the various goods in question. The two concepts are inextricably linked; there is little sense in the idea of human rights entitlements without the corresponding notion of obligation. Each human being who possesses the necessary psychological competencies is both a *rights holder* and a *duty bearer*. The ground for rights claims resides in the nature of human beings and the fact that to live a dignified life, people require a number of goods and services. From this perspective, the only variables of ethical relevance are basic human needs, conditions, and interests, while such factors as professional group, culture, ethnicity, gender, or sexual orientation are deemed irrelevant.

Forensic and correctional clinicians have their professional roots in caring or helping professions and are subject to the social norms and ethical codes of these groups. However, they also work in correctional or forensic mental health settings and as such are subject to the social norms in these settings. One set of norms (or professional code) determines the kinds of actions and practices that are acceptable for clinicians working with individuals who have committed *crimes* while the other spells out what constitutes competent professional practice with *mental health* or therapy clients. The two sets of norms can result in an ethical conflict, where clinicians are torn between wanting to safeguard the interests of the community while also helping individuals to live more fulfilling lives. This conflict of roles is known as the *dual relationship problem* and generates many of the significant ethical problems evident in offending practice (Ward, 2013). It seems that the only solution is to go deeper, to ethical norms that underpin both criminal justice and mental health cultures and their associated roles and practices. With its dual aims of risk reduction and well-being enhancement, the GLM is well placed to address this problem if it has additional ethical support from human rights ideas and the associated concept of dignity.

Strength-based approaches to working with individuals, such as the Good Lives Model (Ward & Maruna, 2007), have ethical advantages over purely risk-oriented approaches. Providing individuals with the core skills and resources required to function in ways that reflect their dignity is likely to both promote their capacity to achieve good lives and reduce their risk to others (Ward & Maruna, 2007; Ward & Gannon, 2006). Furthermore, treatment modules such as empathy training, cognitive skills, understanding the offense process, social skills and intimacy training, and emotional regulation are directly concerned with improving individuals' abilities to accurately infer, respond to, and appreciate the experiences and needs of others. Developing the capabilities to improve the quality of their own lives and to respect those of others will necessarily involve recognition of the freedom and well-being of other people—in essence, acknowledge their human rights. The two components of human rights of *entitlements* and *obligations* correspond well to the two primary goals of the GLM: risk reduction (i.e., acknowledgment of other peoples' rights to freedom of movement, etc.) and well-being enhancement (i.e., entitlements to primary goods and means of securing them). In addition, the dual relationship problem is less likely to derail practice as clinicians seek to help people live better lives and reduce the chances they will harm others in the future. Both professional roles of care provider and community protector are explicitly incorporated within the GLM and boost its advantage over purely risk-oriented approaches to rehabilitation.

Human rights and their translation into specific obligations and entitlements resonates with the well-being and risk management requirements of the GLM and the view of human nature this expresses. The function of these ethical concepts and norms is to protect the well-being and freedom aspects of effective agency.

1.4 Practice Framework Level Two: Knowledge-Related Assumptions of the Good Lives Model

The core values and principles of the good lives model practice framework constrain the formulation of its knowledge-related assumptions. The GLM conceptualizes offending behavior in natural and humanistic terms. Human beings are naturally viewed as goal directed. Thus, the GLM proposes that all meaningful human actions represent attempts to secure primary human goods (i.e., experiences, states of being, and activities sought for their own sake). A major theoretical commitment of the GLM is its view of human beings as embodied, embedded, extended, and enactive. We will now describe these features in greater depth.

1.4.1 An Enactive Conception of Agency

Agency consists of a cluster of cognitive and motivational capacities that enable individuals to formulate goals and use them to actively control aspects of their own behavior and to change features of environments in accordance with their plans. Human beings seek to *enact* their goals and thereby modify aspects of themselves and their environments in ways consistent with those goals. Agency always involves a driver with decision-making abilities, goals that stipulate desired outcomes, and actions that carry out these goals. In more complex forms of agency, goals are hierarchically organized into plans, and individuals can reflect on their problem-solving strategies and modify them, if necessary. All agency works by way of information feedback where goals and actions are modified depending on their success or failure.

According to Tomasello (2022), modern human beings possess four types of agency, which help them to adapt to unpredictable and changeable environments. The four types of agency are: (1) *goal-directed agency*, responsible for making simple choices when confronted with immediate problems; (2) *intentional agency*, enabling human beings to construct plans and think of the possible consequences of their actions in more considered ways; (3) *rational agency,* where individuals are able to reflect on the reasons for and against specific plans, anticipate possible barriers, and come up ways of countering obstacles; and (4) *normative agency,* a uniquely human capacity to engage with normative social institutions and act in morally accountable ways.

Each form of agency is embodied within a living, complex dynamic system (a human being), which actively responds to its environment in a goal-directed manner. That is, organisms *enact* their goals onto the environment. While human beings have retained the capacities of animals (e.g., small mammals and great apes), they have also developed abilities that are unique to them, primarily as a function of their social cooperativeness and greater degree of self-reflection (e.g., normative agency). These capacities include being able to

- Engage in basic goal-directed behavior.
- Inhibit responses and choose safe options when under threat.
- Form, implement, and monitor the effectiveness of plans.
- Grasp the perspective of other people and factor this information into planning.
- Anticipate the possible outcomes of different decisions and choose the best option.
- Deliberately reflect on the methods used to generate knowledge and systematically improve them by error-reduction strategies; and
- Create and engage in cooperative social enterprises and form social agencies, such as institutions, which are partly shaped by individual agents, and which in turn shape them.

According to the *enactive* view of agency, in order to function adequately in typically encountered social and physical environments, individuals need to acquire the essential features of agency listed above. If the process of acquiring these agency-related competencies is compromised or impaired in some way, psychological and/or social problems are likely to occur. Because individuals are embodied and embedded in their environment, the primary cause of agency impairments could be social/cultural, biological, or psychological in nature. The goal-directed nature of complex systems and the flexible ability to control their own activities and actions generate the capacity for agency and a sense of identity (Maiese, 2022). In human beings, social and cultural institutions play an especially significant role in the development of knowledge, skills, and plans for living.

As dynamic adaptive systems, human beings exist in relation to specific environments or contexts to which they respond and shape in ways that increase their chances of survival, enhancement, or (ideally) flourishing. The mind is, in part, *extended* into the social, technological, and cultural environment. Cultural resources (e.g., language, norms, institutions, practices, etc.) are simply the contextual aspects of human beings' relationship to their social environment.

Behavior is rarely random and can typically be understood in terms of benefits, environmental constraints, internal resources, and states. Human beings have several innate motivational systems and cognitive, behavioral, and physiological capacities that have been designed to solve different adaptive problems (Aunger & Curtis, 2015). In proximal terms, these systems address a range of environmental challenges, which individuals address utilizing internal (e.g., skills, knowledge, capacities) and external resources (e.g., opportunities, social supports, education, work) acquired during their development and throughout their lives. The achievement of adaptive outcomes (i.e., reasonable levels of well-being) depends on having all of these needs met to at least a minimal degree (Alexandrova, 2017).

In essence, the enactivist conception of agency:

1. Views the mind and persons as embodied, embedded, extended, goal-directed, and constituted of a nested set of systems (physiological, affective, cognitive, social, cultural, etc.)
2. Explicitly states that human beings have a number of inherited motivational systems, which are translated into action plans by a flexible set of cognitive capacities
3. Argues that human agency is underpinned by emotional and core cognitive capacities, and high-level cognitive abilities that help them to construct and implement good lives plans and
4. Appreciates the pervasive role of social and cultural institutions in the scaffolding of individual and group planning

The enactive conception of agency underpins the GLM's assumption that human beings actively seek to achieve primary human goods via the construction of good lives plans and their associated goals (Dent & Ward, 2022). This view is strongly supported by contemporary scientific theories and empirical findings from evolutionary biology, cognitive neuroscience, anthropology, philosophy of science, psychopathology, and developmental psychology (Del Giudice, 2023; Gallagher, 2023; Gibbs, 2006; Maiese, 2022; Tomasello, 2022). From these perspectives, all living organisms are considered to be agents of some kind.

1.4.2 Critique and Reformulation of the Concept of Dynamic Risk Factors

An enactive conception of agency can help researchers and practitioners deconstruct dynamic risk factors (DRF) and, by doing so, reveal their biological, psychological, cultural, and social/societal components. Furthermore, demonstrating links between impairments in the capacities underpinning agency and DRF helps to clarify why individuals commit crimes and what kind of GLM-oriented good lives plan is required to facilitate desistance from crime.

To understand the need to conceptually deconstruct DRFs when formulating cases, it is first necessary to grasp their limitations as causal or theoretical concepts (Heffernan et al., 2019; Ward & Fortune, 2016). The literature indicates that researchers and clinicians tend to view dynamic risk factors as potential causes of crimes, such as sexual offending (Mann et al., 2010; Ward, 2014). However, DRFs were initially identified to help practitioners assess the risk of recidivism and to classify individuals for the purpose of prison management and resource allocation (Bonta & Andrews, 2017). The additional decision to rely on them for explanatory and treatment targeting purposes came later. This move may have been a mistake, as there are serious conceptual problems with the theory behind DRFs that make them unsuitable for any explanatory and treatment guidance role (Ward & Beech, 2015; Ward & Fortune, 2016). In brief, they are *composite or hybrid concepts* that contain very different types of psychological variables, ranging from causal (e.g., social skill deficits) to mental state factors (e.g., loneliness). Each type of factor class typically contains numerous, sometimes theoretically competing, ideas. For example, there are several possible causes "hidden" in the DRF of emotional congruence, which in turn is only one possible causal factor within the larger class of relational problems (Ward & Fortune, 2016). Because DRFs are essentially risk predictors, in part they are normatively (based on moral and ethical values) defined and arguably do not track distinct causal processes (Cording et al., 2016). Of concern, the same types of theoretical issues also apply to the concept of protective factors, which are currently a major focus of researchers and clinicians in the sexual offending area (Cording et al., 2016; de Vries Robbé et al., 2015; Ward, 2017).

There is a conceptual problem in the lack of causal specificity for the DRF of intimacy deficits in the sexual offending area (Mann et al., 2010; Thornton, 2013). Individuals exhibiting intimacy or relationship problems might have difficulties maintaining and establishing intimate relationships with adults for several distinct reasons, all of which can be incorporated within the agent-action-context schema of the enactivist conception of human functioning. For example:

- They could consider children as sources of reward and more likely to provide them with love, sexual pleasure, and care. It follows that they might seek out opportunities for interpersonal engagement with children (agent beliefs).
- They may view adults as threats and employ avoidance strategies to manage their fear and anxiety, including seeking contact with children (actions).
- Individuals might view the world in general as dangerous and unpredictable, which might lead them to seek solace in the innocence of children and their world (agent beliefs and actions).
- They believe that children are competent sexual agents who can make informed decisions about engaging in sex with adults (agent beliefs).
- They may lack the necessary communication and social skills to maintain relationships with adults and feel emotionally safer with children (agent competences and actions).

- They might find it difficult to adopt another person's perspective and find adult relationships confusing (agent skill).
- They could hold hostile attitudes toward women and believe they are likely to harm them in some way (agent beliefs).
- They may lack the capacity to soothe themselves and, to manage negative physiological arousal, have sex with children (agent actions).
- They might have deviant sexual preferences directed toward children and consequently are not motivated to form intimate relationships with adults (agent values).
- They could belong to social networks that support sexual offending attitudes and share information and videos involving sex with children or work in roles that give them access to children (agent context).

Each item on this list of possible causes originates in distinct constituents of agency and their associated functional systems. For example, cultural norms specify what types of romantic relationship are appropriate, prescribe gender roles, and state how people should act within relationships. From a social perspective, individuals acquire specific interpersonal styles based on their learning history and personality. In addition, contextual factors influence the degree of support they are likely to receive from other people and their status within the community, much of which they have no significant control over. From a first-person agential stance, the experience of fear and loneliness and their origins in core beliefs and attitudes is partly learned through social experience and exposure to family and peer groups. However, learning deficits may also create difficulties for individuals in sustaining attention, forming beliefs, developing coherent plans, and navigating daily life. These kinds of impairments arguably occur at the sub-personal level of psychological functioning and are more likely to occur across different cultural contexts. At a neuropsychological level, neurotransmitters, and hormones like oxytocin, vasopressin, and serotonin, are necessary for normal personal and social functioning. Dysregulation in these systems can create maladaptive behavioral cascades and ultimately, psychological and social problems (e.g., crime, intimacy deficits, etc). Finally, biological variables—high levels of physiological arousal, poor health, physical disabilities —can contribute to both impaired agential functioning, social stigmatization, and rejection.

From a GLM perspective, DRFs reflect problems in the way individuals formulate goals, construct plans, and go about implementing them in specific contexts. In other words, DRFs are best understood as proxies or signal devices (see Chap. 2) for impairments in the capacities underlying agency and relevant contexts that result in behavior that is harmful and/or illegal. They provide descriptions of problems typically observed in individuals who persistently offend and, in their environments, point to areas of vulnerability rather than constituting specific causes of offending. That is, DRFs are summaries of possible causal factors, contextual features, and mental state variables that can be deconstructed to reveal their biological, psychological, social, and cultural components. They are best viewed as signaling devices (see Chap. 2) that highlight areas of concern for the community, clinicians, and often individuals who commit offenses. By viewing them as signaling impairments in the internal capacities and environmental resources, we have linked them to both the enactive conception of the mind and core motivational systems.

1.4.3 Primary Human Goods and Secondary Goods (Means)

The research evidence from multiple disciplines suggests that human beings have a number of innate motivational systems and cognitive, behavioral, and physiological capacities that have been designed to solve different adaptive problems, including caregiving, understanding other people, or seeking status (Aunger & Curtis, 2015; Cummins, 1996; Diener et al., 2002; Emmons, 1999; Gallagher, 2023; Tomasello, 2022). In proximal terms, these systems address a range of environmental challenges, which individuals approach using internal (e.g., skills, knowledge, capacities) and external resources (e.g., opportunities, social supports, education, work) acquired during their development and throughout their lives. The achievement of adaptive outcomes (i.e., reasonable levels of well-being) depends on having all these needs met at least to a minimal degree (Alexandrova, 2017; Ward & Maruna, 2007). This pluralistic conception of human motivation and its relationship to behavior is best described:

> In sum, motivational systems set the goals of behavior and monitor causes of success and failure in the pursuit of those goals. Motivational systems affect behavior indirectly by triggering emotions, which in turn coordinate adaptive suites of physiological, cognitive, and behavioral responses (De Giudice 2018, p.37).

Primary Human Goods (PHGs) derive from core motivational systems and serve as practice-friendly formulations of these concepts (for more details on motivational systems and their relationship to PHG, see Chap. 2). Essentially, PHGs are actions, states of affairs, characteristics, experiences, and states of mind that are beneficial to human beings and sought for their own sake rather than as a means to a more fundamental end (Ward, 2002a, 2002b; Ward & Marshall, 2004). This means that they have intrinsic value (are meaningful and valuable in and of themselves) and represent fundamental purposes and ultimate ends of human behavior.

It should be noted that PHGs within the GLM are conceptualized differently from goals. PHGs are higher-order factors that are realized through the formulation and implementation of goals. As such, PHGs oversee or envelop personal goals. PHGs are ever constant, are considered universal to all human beings, and can be sought and realized through ongoing subjective goal setting (Alexandrova, 2017; Arnhart, 1998). They are operationalized through goals that may be short term, long term, or ever-lasting. In short, goals represent individuals' subjective desires to achieve universal PHGs. In therapeutic practice, the responsivity principle requires that PHGs are operationalized—made concrete—for clients through the formulation of goals, whether these are life goals or more discrete, concrete goals. Goals are a necessary way for people to devise pathways and opportunities to achieve PHGs.

Individuals often have clear ideas about what their goals are, and (depending on the type of goal, the desired outcome, or the people involved) the relationship between goals and PHGs is generally obvious.

The next important concept includes *secondary human goods* (means). Ward (2010) discusses the notion of instrumental goods, which specify ways of achieving primary goods. It may be simpler to understand instrumental goods as the *means* (e.g., strategies and concrete behaviors) associated with a particular good. The notion of means is particularly important when it comes to applying the GLM to offending behavior, as a major reason individuals commit offenses may be because they are pursuing PHGs in problematic and ultimately destructive ways: "all human actions are arguably linked to the seeking of human goods, including the pursuit of anti-social goals" (Ward, 2002b, p. 174). This point emphasizes the distinction between the seeking of PHGs (which are legitimate, valid, and worthwhile) and the means by which they are sought (which, in the case of offending behavior, is problematic and harmful). Simply put, what the individual is seeking at a general level is acceptable, but the way they are going about it is not.

Based on past and current cross-cultural and cross-discipline research, there are 11 PHGs. It should be noted that these PHGs have emerged from thorough analysis of research findings related to personal strivings and the pursuit of healthy lives characterized by high levels of well-being (Alexandrova, 2017; Aunger & Curtis, 2015; Del Giudice, 2023). Given this, the GLM and its account of PHGs may be considered an evolving theory, always open to adaptation, refinement, and development, based on the ever-evolving nature of world knowledge and empirical research. The 11 PHGs are:

- Life
- Knowledge
- Mastery in play
- Mastery in work
- Agency
- Inner peace
- Relatedness
- Community
- Spirituality
- States of happiness and pleasure
- Creativity

In no particular order, the full definitions of the PHGs are presented below.

Life The primary human good of *life* incorporates all the physical needs and factors that are important for healthy living and physical functioning: food, water, shelter, a physically healthy body, and so on. Essentially, optimal fulfillment of this good requires not only that the individual's basic needs for survival are met but that beyond this, their physical health and well-being needs are met. The good of *life* also requires that the person's living circumstances are adequate and suited to their needs. Ideal fulfillment of this good would mean that the person presents as a physically healthy person whose physical functioning and living circumstances are of a high standard.

The seeking of this good may result in a range of activities, such as gaining secure and stable accommodation, engaging in physical exercise or sports, being diet conscious, preparing healthy meals, managing one's own finances to ensure basic needs are met, and managing specific health problems, like allergies or high blood pressure. Problematic ways of seeking the PHG of *life* could be stealing in order to buy food or pay rent.

Knowledge The primary human good of *knowledge* is not concerned with IQ or how smart someone is, rather knowledge-seeking and acquisition consider how well informed an individual is about things that are important to them. This PHG is based on the notion that people are fundamentally curious beings who possess the innate desire to understand aspects of themselves, their environments, and/or other people. The good of knowledge satisfies this need and includes acquiring wisdom or information, including facts, theories, or ideas that can be used to answer questions about areas of interest. For some people, the good of knowledge might be achieved by knowing a great deal about one or a few topics of interest (depth of knowledge). For others, it may be achieved by having limited knowledge about many diverse things (breadth of knowledge). An individual may also seek knowledge via both paths.

Knowledge-related activities and behaviors might include asking questions, studying at university or school, participating in training, vocational pursuits, self-study activities, belonging to a discussion group, or taking lessons to acquire a new skill. Problematic ways of seeking and displaying knowledge include researching alarm systems or reading profiling books to plan crimes and reduce the chances of being caught.

Mastery in Play Human beings seek to enjoy and excel at a range of recreational pursuits that may or may not be structured into games or events. This good refers to the desire to engage in leisure or fun activities that provide the person with a sense of pride, achievement, satisfaction, or skill development. The underlying idea of the PHG of *play* involves both engaging in activities for the purpose of enjoyment, as well as achieving mastery in the area. This good is likely to have both an intrinsic value (accomplishment for the sake of it, i.e., for personal enjoyment) and an instrumental value (accomplishment for a specific purpose, i.e., to win a competition, move up to the next grade/level, or to achieve greater physical fitness). It must be matched to an individual's personal set of skills, interests, preferences, and desires.

Play-related activities and behaviors may include participating in competitive or social teams, individual sporting competitions, hobbies, socializing with friends, organized discussion groups like movie or book clubs. A problematic way of seeking mastery in play is the implementation of coercive sexual practices involving domination role play.

Mastery in Work This good refers to one's need to be meaningfully employed in a role that provides mastery experiences and challenges matched to the person's level of functioning. Mastery *in work* refers to the desire to engage in work that provides the person with a sense of pride, achievement, satisfaction and/or skill development. Meaningful employment will have both an intrinsic value (accomplishment for the sake of it, i.e., for personal fulfillment) and an instrumental value (accomplishment for a specific purpose, i.e., a promotion, greater responsibility, or salary increase). It must also be matched to an individual's personal set of skills, interests, preferences, and desires.

Work-related activities may include participating in meaningful paid employment, meaningful volunteer work, self-employment, undergoing apprenticeships and professional development courses. Problematic ways of seeking mastery at work might include using computing skills to groom children for sexual exploitation or commit fraud.

Agency This PHG refers to human beings' desire to formulate their own goals and seek ways to realize them in actions and activities of their own choice. It accommodates an adult's need for autonomy, self-directedness, personal power, control, and mastery and concerns the individual's ability to act in a way that produces a specific and desired outcome. *Agency* also refers to the desire to make up one's own mind and function as an independent being at least to some minimal degree without interference from others (moderated by cultural and social norms of course). The PHG of agency encompasses the desire to stand on one's own two feet, to be able to pursue things an individual values most, and to shape their lives in ways that are consistent with their deepest values and concerns.

Agency-relevant activities and behaviors include engaging in assertive actions (asserting oneself and one's needs), self-reflection, or achieving financial independence. Problematic means of seeking agency might be attempts to mentally or physically injure, dominate, control, or manipulate others.

Inner Peace The primary human good of *inner peace* refers to emotional self-regulation, the ability to achieve a state of emotional balance, and the need for emotional competence. Emotional competence is basically the application of self-regulation processes to the emotional domain. It includes such skills as awareness and understanding of one's own emotional state, the ability to express how we feel, the capacity to identify other peoples' emotions, the capacity to respond empathically to other people, and the ability to manage aversive emotions through adaptive strategies.

Relevant activities and behaviors for the PHG of inner peace may include a combination of activities such as achieving a balanced lifestyle, building positive relationships with others, learning emotional control and other self-regulation skills, talking to others, meditation, counseling, or physical exercise. These activities can reduce emotional stress and psychological turmoil, while enabling the person to interact with others in an emotionally competent way, thereby increasing psychological well-being. Problematic ways of seeking inner peace might be the use of drugs or coercive sex to escape from aversive affective states.

Relatedness The good of *relatedness* stems from the natural desire of human beings to establish warm affectionate bonds with other people, ranging from romantic relationships to intimate family relationships and platonic yet close friendships—essentially, to love and be loved. As such, this PHG refers to the close, caring, mutual relationships that adults establish with an intimate partner, family members, and close friends. Activities that constitute the good of relatedness include personal disclosure, communication, support, sexual activity, physical contact, honesty, spending time together, sharing interests, mutual emotional caring, equality, and so on.

Seeking the PHG of relatedness may produce a range of results centered on relationships, including all types of adult intimate romantic relationships, close family relationships, or very close friendships. Specifically, instrumental goods are likely to include establishing and maintaining intimate or romantic relationships, establishing and maintaining friendships with others, spending time with family, and having and parenting children. Problematic ways of seeking relatedness needs might be through the sexual abuse of children or engaging in voyeuristic activities.

Community The primary good of *community* refers to the desire human beings have to belong to social groups or to feel connected to groups that reflect their interests, concerns, and values. It is the sense of being part of a wider social and/or cultural network, to feel one is contributing to a larger social unit, and to be able to rely on this larger group to meet one's own needs.

Community-related activities and behaviors may include belonging to social service groups or special interest groups (e.g., a political party, a sporting club, a craft group, book club, nature/wildlife group, or religious affiliations), engaging in volunteer work, or being part of a neighborhood group or school activity. Problematic approaches to finding a sense of community include joining a gang that is heavily involved in criminal activities or participating in a pedophilic online network.

Spirituality The primary good of *spirituality* refers to the desire discover a sense of meaning and purpose in life and achieve the overall experience of being content and satisfied with one's life. This could involve seeking religious truths and affiliation, a spiritual connection with a transcendent being or reality, or simply the experience of being part of a wider whole. In short, the PHG of spirituality refers to the broad sense of purpose and direction in an individual's life and relates to the overall feeling of happiness and contentedness that emerges from understanding one's involvement with the world around them.

Spirituality-related activities and behaviors may include belonging to a church, studying philosophy, joining an environmental organization, having a clear vision or plan for one's future and life direction, or living one's life according to a particular set of values (such as ethical behaviors and nonviolence). An example of problematic relationship involving the PHG of spirituality is the sexual abuse of children within spiritual or religious contexts. Sometimes, in these situations individuals are seeking what they perceive as religiously justified sexual relationships with children.

States of Happiness and Pleasure[2] This primary human good refers to a positive state of being (feeling good in the here and now) and includes a range of feelings and sensations like joy, merriment, delight, elation, and hedonic pleasure, which is essentially healthy self-indulgence and gratification. It is often implicated in activities that bring about feelings of enjoyment, deep satisfaction, and excitement. This is different from overarching life contentment and happiness characterized by overall well-being, which emerges from the degree to which all the primary goods have been achieved.

Activities and behaviors related to the PHG of happiness and pleasure may include establishing relationships that result in pleasure and joy, enjoyment of food, getting a massage, engaging in sexual activity, thrill-seeking activities, or participation in sports or recreational activities, and so on. In all cases, the goal is largely a feeling of joy, pleasure, and gratification. A problematic way of seeking pleasure is through masochistic practices with a non-consenting person.

Creativity The primary human good of *creativity* refers to a desire for novelty, innovation, and individuality in one's life. It may be reflected in the experience of doing things differently, being engaged in a specific type of activity that results in an artistic output, or perhaps producing a novel product of some kind. Creativity does not require that an individual be artistic in a traditional sense, as it may be implicated in a range of everyday activities; creativity is essentially the expression of oneself through alternative forms of activity.

Activities and behaviors related to creativity may include work, parenting, gardening, woodwork, painting, attending art exhibitions, solving problems, devising new methods of doing something, playing a musical instrument, etc. Creativity may also be expressed in how we dress and present ourselves (e.g., personal image, tattoos, piercing, etc.) or how we set up our home, including the colors, fabrics, furniture we select. A problematic way of seeking creativity is through using children as objects of sexual self-expression and manipulation.

While all 11 of the above PHGs typically need to be present to some degree in every individuals' good lives plans if they are to experience satisfactory levels of well-being, they may vary in their respective ratings of the importance of each good. For some people, the primary good of knowledge is most highly prized, while others might value personal relationships or work more highly. The most highly weighted PHG and its translation into secondary goods or means is what gives individuals a sense of purpose and meaning. It is closely aligned with what we call *practical identity*, that is, a description under which individuals find aspects of themselves and their lives valuable (Korsgaard, 2009). Examples of practical

[2] Readers may note that past GLM publications have referred to this PHG as either Happiness or Pleasure. The refinement of the labeling and definition of this PHG in this text serves to amalgamate the key points to be emphasized from previous publications. That is, that this PHG is concerned with *states* of happiness and pleasure, hence the adjustment in its reference title. The specific reasons for this change are discussed in detail later in this chapter.

identities include a university professor working in service of the PHG of knowledge or a car mechanic whose core value is mastery at work. What is especially pertinent for therapists is that if a person is unable to find ways of achieving their most highly weighted PHG, they are likely to feel their lives lack meaning. In such cases, people commonly speak of feeling empty, flat, without purpose, depressed, or grief stricken. The weightings of PHGs may also vary over the course of individuals' lives in response to their changing biological, psychological, and social circumstances.

1.4.4 Good Lives Plans: How and When Things Go Wrong

According to the GLM, people offend because they are attempting to secure some kind of valued outcome in their life. As such, offending is essentially the product of a desire for something that is inherently human and normal, but the desire or goal manifests itself in harmful and antisocial behaviors due to a range of deficits within the individual and his environment (Laws & Ward, 2011). Essentially, these deficits prevent individuals from securing their desired ends in prosocial and sustainable ways, thus requiring them to resort to inappropriate and damaging means (i.e., offending).

There are several problems that can occur in the way people live their lives (i.e., lifestyle) or the life plan they have mentally constructed. A *way of living* refers to how a person is currently living their lives in terms of daily activities, functioning, or behaviors and generally represents a lifestyle that reflects certain individual values and attitudes. A *life plan* refers to how a person plans (either implicitly or explicitly) to live their lives now and in the future. Sometimes, the way people actually live their lives can be very different from the way they intended (or planned) to do so. According to Ward (2002; Ward & Fisher, 2006), there are four primary types of problems that can be evident in a person's way of living or life plan: scope, capacity, appropriateness of means, and coherence.

Scope The first problem with ways of living and life plans concerns their degree of scope. When a person either fails to strive for or secure (at some level) each of the 11 basic goods, their good life plan is considered to lack scope. A lack of scope is likely to lead to one or a combination of problems, including physiological dysfunction, psychological distress leading to mental health problems, or social maladjustment (Ward, 2002), all of which will invariably lead to a decrease in one's overall life happiness. Problems in scope can simply be caused by a disinterest in some goods; however, a lack of scope is usually caused by problems in capacity. For example, lack of interpersonal skills or distrust of others can cause problems in securing the goods of relatedness and community and may create difficulties at work (excellence at work), reduce engagement in leisure activities involving others (excellence in play), and cause an overall neglect of the socially oriented PHGs. This person's life would be said to lack scope.

Capacity The second problem with ways of living and life plans concerns capacity. This essentially assesses the person's strengths and weaknesses. There are two types of capacities to consider, *internal capacity* and *external capacity*. Internal capacity refers to factors internal to individuals, such as skill level, mental health, attitudes, and beliefs. Internal factors can be broadly psychological (e.g., beliefs, motivation, attitudes, mental health), cognitive (the individual's level of knowledge or mental ability), behavioral (cognitive or psychological factors that result in behaviors which limit or enhance the individual's abilities and opportunities), and physical (the person's level of health and wellness impacting functioning and abilities). Positive and beneficial capacities can be referred to as internal strengths. Problems with internal capacity are referred to as internal obstacles and basically represent weaknesses (for example, depression, negative beliefs about the trustworthiness of women, or pro-criminal attitudes). It may be that an individual lacks the internal conditions necessary to secure certain goods, and as such, the enhancement or acquiring of particular skills or internal conditions should be a focus of treatment. For instance, individuals wishing to emphasize the good of mastery in work, however, may lack the skills to gain the type of work that they believe will give them sense of achievement and fulfillment. The focus of intervention should not be to get the person a job but to help them equip themselves with the skills necessary to secure the job that will bring the fulfillment they seek.

In contrast, external capacity relates to those conditions or contexts external to the individual (e.g., environmental factors, social supports, employment opportunities, access to education, etc.), which are needed to attain PHGs and their associated goals. Therefore, PHG-supportive external factors can be thought of as external strengths. Problems with external capacity are referred to as external obstacles or weaknesses. To illustrate, an individual may want to become an artist. This is the goal, but the good sought may be mastery in work, mastery in play, or creativity. However, because they live in a geographically isolated location (external obstacle) there are no courses nearby that they can enroll in. Internal and external obstacles or weaknesses can therefore govern the means used to reach this goal. In the above example, the external obstacle of geographical isolation may lead the individual to buy an art book and teach themselves—this assumes the presence of internal strengths such as motivation, self-belief, literacy skills, etc. Alternatively, the individual may just resolve to give up (due to internal weaknesses, such as lack of motivation, poor self-confidence and belief, poor literacy skills), therefore allowing the goal and associated goods to go unfulfilled. This may, in turn, lead to problems in scope.

Means The third problem concerns the appropriateness of means and essentially refers to the behaviors or strategies people use to secure PHGs or their associated goals. PHGs can be sought in any number of ways, and sometimes in ways that hinder individuals' chances of either securing the good successfully or receiving the true benefit of the good. Problems in means are often caused by problems in capacity. When a person lacks strengths, but has internal and external weaknesses, they are more likely to engage in problematic behaviors in a dysfunctional attempt at securing goals and PHGs.

For example, a depressed person may seek the PHG of inner peace, but has poor interpersonal skills (internal deficit), minimal social supports (external obstacle), and doesn't know how to seek out or access psychological services (internal deficit). As a result, their means for securing the PHG of inner peace is through withdrawing emotionally from others and engaging in substance abuse. However, substance abuse and emotional withdrawal are inappropriate means, as they end up compounding the emotional turmoil when the person becomes lonely, feels rejected, experiences relationship breakdowns, suffers poor health and physical functioning, and finally runs into job loss and financial problems. Therefore, the problematic means (caused by problems in capacity) by which the individual is seeking this good, results in the good not being properly secured and the person's needs unfulfilled. Contrary to what they might have hoped for, the person is likely to experience a further decrease in levels of happiness due to their frustrated efforts.

Coherence and Conflict The final problem with ways of living and good life plans involves incoherence or conflict of goods. It is important that in each person's life, PHGs are at least roughly ordered and coherently related to each other. Ward (2002) argues that a life lacking in coherence is likely to lead to frustration and harm to the individual concerned and may also lead to a life lacking in overall sense of purpose and meaning. Ward and Stewart (2003) state that there are two types of coherence problems: *horizontal coherence* and *vertical coherence*.

Horizontal coherence refers to the extent to which goods are explicitly related to each other in a mutually consistent and enabling way. That is, PHGs need to be sought and acquired in ways that are prosocial and personally meaningful, so as not to cause problems in the seeking of other goods and creating horizontal conflict. Essentially, goods need to complement each other or exist harmoniously alongside one another, rather than being antagonistic or conflicting. For instance, a person may be committed to securing the primary good of relatedness through a romantic relationship; however, they may also be committed to securing the good of agency. Though the two PHGs may be equally important, they may also conflict due to the type of means used; the individual wants to feel close and secure with someone but behaves oppressively and abusively so as to feel autonomous, powerful, and in control. The problem is that the means to seek the PHG of agency negates the person's ability to secure the PHG of relatedness, because people end up not liking the person and feel threatened by them. This type of conflict between goods is likely to cause relationship problems, the thwarting of the relatedness good, emotional distress, and ultimately, unhappiness. Obviously, the problem lies in seeking certain goods in ways that harm other people while also seeking to be close and connected to people. Conflict between goods can also lead to a lack of scope. Research has found that goal conflict and failure to achieve important personal goals has negative effects on physical well-being (Emmons, 1999).

The second form of coherence—vertical coherence—means that PHGs require hierarchical clarity or ranking in terms of priority and importance. While the GLM specifies that all goods should be sought in each person's life, it does not specify the level of importance assigned to each good. This is an entirely individual process, informed by each person's preferences, skills, likes and dislikes, social norms, and cultural values. Individuals need to understand which goods are most important to them and have the most priority in their life. These priorities should govern the level of investment assigned to each PHG and what activities the individual engages in on a daily basis. Someone who weights the good of relatedness over mastery in work is going to be relatively unhappy if they actually live their life as a single person who works long hours 7 days a week. This situation represents vertical conflict, and an intervention should first identify the discrepancy between what is desirable to the person and what they are actually doing/how they are actually living their life. Second, interventions should motivate and support the person to make changes. It is plausible to argue hierarchical conflict (i.e., a lack of time and investment in prioritized PHGs) causes people to feel unfulfilled in how they live their lives, and leads to a sense of meaninglessness and unhappiness, potentially making people focus on immediate gratification over the fulfillment of long-term life goals (Ward & Stewart, 2003). Criminogenic needs (DRFs) are conceptualized within the GLM as signaling internal or external agency impairments that make it difficult for individuals to secure PHGs in personally meaningful and socially acceptable ways.

In sum, there are a variety of problems that may be evident in people's ways of living and life plans. It should be the aim of rehabilitation to identify what problems exist so that lifestyles and life plans can be addressed to suit each individual's preferences, capabilities, skills, temperament, and opportunities. This would allow them to access goods in prosocial ways that are intrinsically beneficial and meaningful. Finally, because the GLM acknowledges and values the preferences and experience of individuals, intervention is directly aimed at addressing risk areas that are high priority PHGs for those individuals. Ideally, this naturally motivates them to engage in the rehabilitation process, as the focus of intervention is precisely oriented to the things they consider to be of most importance and value.

1.4.5 Pathways to Offending: How PHGs Become Implicated in Offending Behavior

When practitioners understand the nature of a client's functioning in terms of scope, capacity, means, and coherence, they essentially understand the factors that are either helping or inhibiting their attainment of healthy prosocial living and well-being. According to the GLM, offending is basically a person's inappropriate and harmful way of seeking otherwise legitimate goals and PHGs. Perhaps the individual sought to feel in control, powerful, important (PHG agency), intimate (PHG relatedness), or sexually gratified (PHG states of happiness and pleasure) when they committed their criminal acts. Under normal circumstances, these are reasonable goals that almost all adults, regardless of gender or cultural connection, will seek to have or experience at various points in their life. In fact, the pursuit of all 11 PHGs is entirely human and normal. What is unacceptable is the way in which the individuals who offend seek them, for example, by sexually violating, humiliating, and/or harming another person. These strategies represent problematic means, typically underpinned by problems in capacity or skill.

Direct and indirect pathways PHGs can be directly or indirectly implicated in offending behavior, and an individual may have a combination of both direct and indirect pathways with multiple PHGs implicated in offending behavior. These direct and indirect routes correspond to the approach and avoidant pathways identified in the Self-Regulation Model (Ward & Hudson, 2000; Yates & Ward, 2008).

A solid understanding of PHGs' direct and indirect pathways related to an individual's offending behavior is vital in terms of risk management and sound intervention planning. These components of the model are comprehensively explained elsewhere with clear examples (Purvis et al., 2011), therefore focus here is on the role of PHGs in direct and indirect pathways to offending behavior.

In terms of the direct pathway, the person plans and intends to offend as a means (albeit inappropriate) of securing a particular PHG. Specifically, if the means for a good is to offend, then the seeking of that good is deemed to follow a direct pathway to offending. For example, the PHG of agency is likely to be directly implicated in offending behavior for someone who offends for the primary purpose of feeling important, powerful, in control, and respected. It may not be the only PHG directly or indirectly implicated.

Indirect pathways are slightly more complex. In this instance, the person does not have the express intention of offending but rather is focused on achieving a certain PHG through a non-offending means. The problem is that the means is either inappropriate or non-existent (e.g., due to problems in capacity, the person may have no available means for achieving the good, therefore the good goes unsecured, and the related goal unfulfilled). Either way, both the inappropriate means and the lack of means results will thwart the good (an associated goal/s) and increase the pressure to offend. This means that the PHG is essentially unsecured, either by being completely inaccessible or by being secured only temporarily (or minimally) with problematic behaviors, which undermines the true value of the good. The problematic means create a ripple or cascade effect on the person's life. In other words, it makes their life or situation worse, while compounding problems, dissatisfaction, and unhappiness lead them to offend. For example, a person may struggle to achieve emotional equilibrium (inner peace), primarily because they lack core emotional competencies. Pressures at work could increase their drinking, resulting in impaired performance, marital difficulties, and increased drinking that allows disinhibited behavior. Ultimately, this cascade effect might result in intense experiences of anger toward a female employer and culminate in an assault on a female stranger.

Understanding direct and indirect pathways provides practitioners with an understanding of individuals' most significant risk factors and the key intervention targets in need of prioritized intervention. Essentially, the obstacles that drive direct and indirect pathways represent each person's unique risk profile; hence, they support an individualized and tailored approach to intervention by signaling the PHG involved in and problems associated with individuals' good lives plans.

To address problems associated with individuals' offending behavior, treating clinicians and case managers need to help them acquire the necessary skills, attributes, and environments to pursue their goals via alternative, prosocial means. The promotion of PHGs within the GLM approach is at the very core of this behavior change work. Specifically, translating an individual's motivations for offending into an understanding of their dysfunctional approach to seeking of PHGs reveals what the individual values and strives for, even in the face of considerable obstacles.

1.5 Level Three: Intervention Guidelines of the Good Lives Model

With respect to the moral status of individuals who have committed crimes, the good lives practice framework views them as "fellow travelers" or "people like us." Therefore, therapists are encouraged to see clients as sharing the same needs and aspirations as non-offending individuals and to work collaboratively in a nonpunitive and constructive way.

The domain or epistemic niche of the GLM is therapeutic intervention. The primary focus of a good lives framework intervention is an individual's good lives plan, and the adaptive pursuit of primary human goods in their daily lives. Specifically, the aim of intervention is the promotion of primary goods or human needs that, once met, enhance psychological well-being (Ward & Maruna, 2007). Once a person's conceptualization of what constitutes a good life is understood, future-oriented secondary goods aimed at satisfying primary goods in socially acceptable ways are formulated collaboratively and translated into a good lives treatment plan (GLP). Working within a practice framework perspective reminds researchers that a comprehensive intervention plan typically requires the application of other types of practice framework models, such as the RNR model (risk management, prediction, and policy formation domains) or restorative justice (moral domain), each operating within a distinct domain. Each of these models has a different domain of application, and they complement each other rather than being in direct competition.

1.5.1 GLM Practice Implications

There is a range of key practice commitments that flow from the implementation of a GLM framework. We wish to note the six key practice commitments here (Purvis et al., 2011).

GLM six key practice commitments:

1. Manage the balance between promoting PHGs and reducing risk.
2. View individuals who commit offenses as fellow travelers, not moral strangers.
3. The kinds of language associated with GLM interventions should be future-oriented, optimistic, and approach goal focused.
4. Individuals should be viewed holistically and are more than the sum of their risk factors and criminal records.
5. The Risk-Need-Responsivity principles should be nested or embedded within a GLM framework.
6. Consider individuals' strengths, prioritized PHG, and relevant environments; then specify exactly what competencies and resources are required to achieve these goods.

As stated earlier, the goal of effective intervention is risk management and increased well-being. These two goals should be the shared aims of all those involved in the individual's rehabilitation, and the main two contexts within which rehabilitation can and should take place are within both therapy and case management. As stated in practice commitment five, the primary principles of the Risk-Need-Responsivity Model (Bonta & Andrews, 2017) are explicitly incorporated within the GLM. As such, it is a comprehensive and seamless rehabilitation framework (Ward & Maruna, 2007). In brief, high-risk individuals have more problems in their GLP (i.e., typically display all four types of flaws in multiple ways) and require more intervention; intervention should make sure that problems highlighted by criminogenic needs are targeted. In the GLM, the aim is to create capabilities that assist individuals to achieve personal goals rather than simply reduce risk. The responsivity principle is clearly incorporated in the GLM's focus on individuals' personal priorities, abilities, and situation.

With regard to the practice implications of the GLM, the aims of intervention are to assist individuals to acquire knowledge, skills, and competencies to obtain their PHGs in nonharmful and acceptable ways, to overcome flaws in their good life plans, and to reduce and/or manage their risk of recidivism (e.g., Willis et al., 2013). There are two ways risk reduction can occur. First, the establishment of the internal and external capacities needed to achieve a primary good (or more broadly, implement a GLP) in socially acceptable and personally fulfilling ways can directly alter factors indexed by dynamic risk factors (criminogenic needs). For example, learning the skills necessary to become a wood carver will make it easier for someone to develop concentration and emotional regulations skills, thereby reducing impulsivity, a criminogenic need. Second, the reduction of risk can occur indirectly when an individual is strongly motivated to work hard in treatment because of their involvement in projects that personally engage them. For example, an individual might work hard at overcoming their substance abuse problems because they are keen to attend a mechanic vocational course. In actual practice, GLP can impact both directly and indirectly on problems highlighted or signaled by dynamic risk factors.

From a GLM perspective, practice foci are on the core ideas of agency, psychological well-being, and the opportunity to live a different type of life that is personally meaningful and satisfying. At the same time, it addresses risk factors for reoffending (Ward & Stewart, 2003; Yates et al., 2010). An important therapeutic task involves managing the delicate balance between the approach goal of promoting the individual's goods and the avoidance goal of reducing risk. Making mistakes on the side of either goal can lead to undesirable social and personal consequences for the practitioner and the client (Ward & Birgden, 2007). More specifically, simply seeking to enhance the well-being without consideration for his or her level of risk may result in a happy but dangerous individual. Conversely, attempting to manage risk without concern for goods promotion or well-being could lead to punitive practices, as well as disengaged and hostile clients.

The GLM rehabilitation approach can be illustrated using five phases (Laws & Ward, 2011; Ward & Maruna, 2007; Yates & Prescott, 2011; Yates et al., 2010). The first phase of intervention involves identifying the social, psychological, and environmental aspects of offending, including individuals' level of risk and their social, physical, and psychological resources (e.g., substance use, accommodation and financial situation, and personality patterns, such as level of impulsivity) at the time of offending and in the past. The second phase identifies the function of offending-related actions through an exploration of the PHGs directly and indirectly associated with the offending behavior (a backward-looking task). The third phase involves identifying core practical identities (i.e., a description of the person's overarching most heavily weighted primary goods and the way these are embedded within specific roles or activities) and their associated PHGs or values to assist with the development of a life plan (a forward-looking task). Once an individual's conceptualization of what constitutes a good life is understood, future-oriented secondary goods can be identified collaboratively and can assist in achieving their desired PHGs in socially acceptable ways.

The fourth phase involves generating details from the previous phase, including the secondary goods (i.e., means) that will help translate PHGs/values into a way of functioning that results in a good life. This information is used to subsequently develop a good lives plans (GLP). Moreover, it is important to be aware of the context within which the offending behavior occurred and the environments that the individual is likely to be released into. This includes considering the social, psychological, and material resources that will be available to assist them in attaining their primary goals. To do this, it is necessary for the goals to be divided into achievable steps within the associated time frames. Standard goal-setting techniques are relevant here (e.g., setting goals that are specific, measurable, achievable, realistic, and with a time frame).

The fifth phase involves developing a detailed intervention, a good lives plan (GLP) that is comprehensive and incorporates the internal and external conditions required to accomplish the GLP that revolves around an individuals' core goals/values and practical identities. It is crucial to identify specific steps so that the plan can be effectively implemented. This phase must include the required resources/supports necessary to achieve it. It should also be emphasized that the GLP should be driven by the values, goals, and identities of the individual, while the practitioner assists with forming the plan and balancing other considerations such as ethical entitlements of victims and the wider community.

1.5.2 Desistance Factors

The GLM was originally developed as a strength-based model to provide comprehensive guidance to clinicians working with individuals within the criminal justice system. In retrospect, this was a major limitation, as it had relatively little to say about how to work with individuals who (1) receive community-based sentences or (2) have left prison and are now back in the community. Ward and his colleagues explicitly addressed this weakness by integrating desistance research and ideas into the GLM in a book (Laws & Ward, 2011) and several papers (e.g., Ward & Laws, 2010; Willis & Ward, 2024).

The concept of desistance is a complex one and has been defined in numerous ways in the literature (Laws & Ward, 2011). It has been described, for example, as a self-reported complete termination of criminal behavior; a cessation of official citations for criminal behavior; and a marked decrease in the frequency, intensity, and seriousness of criminal behavior. The definition that fits best with the GLM is the view that desistance is not an event, but rather a process replete with lapses, relapses, and recoveries (Maruna, 2001). Desistance research seeks to understand the change processes that are associated with individuals turning away from lives of crime and becoming reintegrated into the community (McNeill et al., 2005). Thus, desistance from criminal behavior is considerably more than simply stopping. As the desistance process advances, there may be intermittency, a combination of pauses, resumptions, indecisiveness, and ambivalence, all of which may finally lead to termination.

It is possible to identify three strands in desistance theory, which stress the importance of maturation, agency, and social relationships (McNeill et al., 2005; Maruna, 2001). Theorists have sometimes contrasted objective desistance factors, e.g., a job or marriage (Glueck & Glueck, 1968; Giordano et al., 2002; Laub & Sampson, 2003), with a subjective sense of meaning arguing for the primacy of one over the other (Weaver & McNeill, 2010). More recent theoretical work has emphasized the interaction between all three sets of desistance factors and the fact that it is in the interfaces between these variables that desistance exerts its effect (Langton & Worling, 2022; McNeill, 2009).

According to the GLM, individuals' core values enable them to capitalize on or create objective events that reflect their practical identity. There is no separation: people constitute themselves through actions, which necessarily involve opportunities and objective events. Because of stress on the importance of the past in fashioning practical identities and the associated socialization and acculturation processes, the GLM also has a strong developmental focus without adopting a fatalistic tone. There is a continual green thread that runs through individuals' lives from the past to the future, linking core values, life plans, identity, and ultimately, meaning. Furthermore, the GLM's stress on agency and the importance of reflectiveness is entirely consistent with desistance theorists' emphasis on turning points (Sampson & Laub, 2005) or critical events that create a sense of crisis in individuals and ultimately prompts them to reevaluate their lives and reconstruct their identities. Identity reconstruction (Maruna, 2001) works through the location of the primary goods that are most important to individuals and an analysis of alternative ways to seek them. Practical identities are constituted by practices and ways of acting in the world and inevitably involve norms that regulate specific actions, dress, habits, and so on. The flexibility of human beings and their natural inclination to seek certain outcomes and to view their lives as meaningful and unified is likely to contribute to self-reflection following crises or turning points.

Desistance theory—with its primary interest on what assists individuals to refrain from committing further crimes once they are released into the community—can extend the reach of the GLM beyond that of correctional treatment programs. Furthermore, the GLM can provide a theoretically grounded and systematic theory to explain why promoting strengths, such as work or good relationships, is desirable and should increase individuals' chances of remaining offense free (Laws & Ward, 2011). It also includes explicit resources to guide and coordinate specific intervention efforts across a wide range of correctional professionals. According to the GLM, individuals' core values enable them to capitalize on or create objective events that reflect their practical identity. Desistance theory adds depth and scope to the social, developmental, and cultural aspects of GLM.

1.6 Conclusion

For those of us working on the front line with complex problems like sexual offending, a number of questions inevitably arise. Why do some individuals commit sexual offenses? How do we keep the community safe and help individuals start the journey back to leading fulfilling and responsible lives? Can they change? What can we do to prevent sexual violence? Individuals who commit sexual offenses have been thought of as monsters (they are not), who cannot change (they can), as completely different to us (untrue), having no redeemable qualities (unlikely), and requiring isolation from our communities (in fact, the opposite is true). If we, as professionals, are serious about making our communities safer, and if we truly want to see individuals finish their sentence and not return to the correctional system, then we need to find a way of working that equips them with the psychological and social tools to live better, more fulfilling, prosocial lives. Society and policymakers are responsible for making this possible for all people as a preventive measure.

The core normative (value), knowledge, and practiced assumptions of the GLM can be incorporated within the overarching enactive concept of human agency with its insistence that human beings are goal-directed organisms whose minds are embodied, embedded within social/cultural environments, and interpersonally and technologically extended (Ward et al., 2024b). Following on from this conception of human functioning, evidence-based practice requires practitioners to take the socially/culturally embedded, extended, and embodied nature of human beings into account in assessment and treatment. Relatedly, it is important to draw an explicit link between crime-related risk factors and well-being concerns in research and practice. This is because individuals are innately motivated to meet a range of basic needs, while crime can be viewed as resulting from problems in the internal and external capacities necessary to achieve goals associated with these needs in prosocial and meaningful ways. Rehabilitation models are best construed as practice frameworks that have core personal, social, and ethical values at their center. Human rights theory and the concept of human dignity provide a strong ethical justification for a combination of risk management and well-being approaches. They explicitly connect the naturalistic and normative aspects of the GLM by virtue of its view of human rights as protective capsules. The GLM is ideally placed to capitalize on both ethical concepts. Primary human goods are underpinned by a suite of motivational systems that human beings share with other primates and which have an evolutionary basis. Dynamic risk factors cannot be directly utilized as explanatory factors and treatment foci. They should only be used as signaling devices and the problems associated with them reformulated in terms of internal and external capacity impairments. Otherwise, they are best understood as predictive tools. Rehabilitation models should incorporate desistance factors such as work, social support, and a sense of meaning, because they facilitate the successful social reentry and integration of persons convicted of crimes. This will enable good live plans to extend the scope of rehabilitation beyond the prison walls and into the community.

The following chapters of this book will unpack the three levels of the GLM practice framework in greater depth and walk the reader through its assessment, practice, and policy guidelines, while illustrating key points with clinical examples.

References

Alexandrova, A. (2017). *A philosophy for the science of well-being*. Oxford University Press.

American Psychological Association, Presidential Task Force on Evidence-Based Practice. (2006). Evidence-based practice in psychology. *American Psychologist, 61*, 271–285. https://doi.org/10.1037/0003-066X.61.4.271

Arnhart, L. (1998). *Darwinian natural right: The biological ethics of human nature*. State University of New York Press.

Aunger, R., & Curtis, V. (2015). *Gaining control: How human behaviour evolved*. Oxford University Press. https://doi.org/10.1176/appi.books.9780890425596

Bonta, J., & Andrews, D. A. (2017). *The psychology of criminal conduct* (6th ed.). Routledge.

Bucknall, T., & Rycroft-Malone, J. (2021). Evidence-based practice: Doing the right thing for patients. In J. Rycroft-Malone & T. Bucknall (Eds.), *Models and frameworks for implementing evidence-based practice: Linking evidence to action* (pp. 1–22). Wiley.

Cording, J. R., Beggs Christofferson, S. M., & Grace, R. C. (2016). Challenges for the theory and application of dynamic risk factors. *Psychology, Crime and Law, 22*(1-2), 84–103.

Cummins, R. A. (1996). The domains of life satisfaction: An attempt to order chaos. *Social Indicators Research, 38*, 303–328.

Del Giudice, M. (2023). A general motivational architecture of human and animal personality. *Neuroscience and Biobehavioral Reviews, 144*. https://doi.org/10.1016/j.neubiorev.2022.104967

Dent, H., & Ward, T. (2022). Emotion and correctional practice: Theoretical foundations of an enactive practice framework. *Aggression and Violent Behavior, 63*. https://doi.org/10.1016/j.avb.2021.101672

de Vries Robbé, M., de Vogel, V., Koster, K., & Bogaerts, S. (2015). Assessing protective factors for sexually violent offending with the SAPROF. *Sexual Abuse: A Journal of Research and Treatment, 27*, 51–70.
Diener, E., Lucas, R. E., & Oishi, S. (2002). Subjective well-being: The science of happiness and life satisfaction. In C. R. Snyder & S. J. Lopez (Eds.), *Handbook of positive psychology* (pp. 63–73). Oxford University Press.
Drisko, J. W., & Grady, M. D. (2019). *Evidence-based practice in clinical social work* (2nd ed.). Springer.
Emmons, R. A. (1999). *The psychology of ultimate concerns*. Guilford Press.
Fazel, S., Hurton, C., Burghart, M., Delisi, M., & Yu, R. Q. (2024). An updated evidence synthesis on the Risk-Need-Responsivity (RNR) model: Umbrella review and commentary. *Journal of Criminal Justice, 92*, 102197. https://doi.org/10.1016/j.jcrimjus.2024.102197
Freeden, M. (1991). *Rights*. University of Minnesota Press.
Gallagher, S. (2023). *Embodied and enactive approaches to cognition*. Cambridge University Press.
Gannon, T., & Ward, T. (2014). Where has all the psychology gone? A critical review of evidence-based psychological practice in correctional settings. *Aggression and Violent Behavior, 19*, 435–436.
Gibbs, R. W. (2006). *Embodiment and cognitive science*. Cambridge University Press.
Giordano, P. C., Cernkovich, S. A., & Rudolph, J. I. (2002). Gender, crime and desistance: Toward a theory of cognitive transformation. *American Journal of Sociology, 107*, 990–1064.
Gewirth, A. (1996). *The community of rights*. The University of Chicago Press.
Glueck, S., & Glueck, E. (1968). *Delinquents and nondelinquents in perspective*. Harvard University Press.
Haig, B. D. (2014). *Investigating the psychological world: Scientific method in the behavioral sciences*. MIT Press.
Haynes, S. C., Barlow, D. H., & Nelson-Gray, R. O. (1999). *The scientist-practitioner: Research and accountability in the age of managed care* (2nd ed.). Pearson.
Heffernan, R., Wegerhoff, D., & Ward, T. (2019). Dynamic risk factors: Conceptualization, measurement, and evidence. *Aggression and Violent Behavior, 48*, 6–16.
Korsgaard, C. M. (2009). *Self-constitution: Agency, identity, and integrity*. Oxford University Press.
Langton, C. M., & Worling, J. R. (Eds.). (2022). *Facilitating desistance from aggression and crime: Theory, research, and strength-based practices*. Wiley-Blackwell.
Laub, J. H., & Sampson, R. J. (2003). *Shared beginnings, divergent lives: Delinquent boys to age 70*. Harvard University Press.
Laws, D. R., & Ward, T. (2011). *Desistance from sexual offending: Alternatives to throwing away the keys*. Guilford Press.
McNeill, F. (2009). What works and what's just? *European Journal of Probation, 1*, 21–40.
McNeill, F., Batchelor, S., Burnett, R., & Knox, J. (2005). *21st century social work. Reducing re-offending: Key practice skills*. Scottish Executive.
Maiese, M. (2022). *Autonomy, enactivism and mental disorder: A philosophical account*. Routledge.
Mann, R. E., Hanson, R. K., & Thornton, D. (2010). Assessing risk for sexual recidivism: Some proposals on the nature of psychologically meaningful risk factors. *Sexual Abuse: A Journal of Research and Treatment, 22*, 191–217. https://doi.org/10.1177/1079063210366039
Maruna, S. (2001). *Making good: How ex-convicts reform and rebuild their lives*. American Psychological Association.
Nathan, M. J. (2021). *Black boxes: How science turns ignorance into knowledge*. Oxford University Press.
Orend, B. (2002). *Human rights: Concept and context*. Broadview.
Purvis, M., Ward, T., & Willis, G. (2011). The good lives model in practice: Offense pathways and case management. *European Journal of Probation, 3*, 4–28.
Sackett, D. L., Straus, S. E., Richardson, W. S., Rosenberg, W., & Haynes, R. B. (2000). *Evidence based medicine: How to practice and teach EBM*. Churchill Livingstone.

Sampson, R. J., & Laub, J. H. (2005). Alife-course view of the development of crime. *Annals of the American Academy of Political and Social Sciences, 602*, 12–45.

Satterfield, J. M., Spring, B., Brownson, R. C., Mullen, E. J., Newhouse, R. P., Walker, B. B., & Whitlock, E. P. (2009). Toward a transdisciplinary model of evidence-based practice. *The Milbank Quarterly, 87*(2), 368–390. https://doi.org/10.1111/j.1468-0009.2009.00561.x

Shapiro, M. B. (1979). Assessment interviewing in clinical psychology. *British Journal of Social and Clinical Psychology, 18*, 211–218. https://doi.org/10.1111/j.2044-8260.1979.tb00329.x

Spring, B., & Neville, K. (2011). Evidence-based practice in clinical psychology. In D. H. Barlow (Ed.), *The Oxford handbook of clinical psychology* (pp. 128–149). Oxford University Press.

Tomasello, M. (2022). *The evolution of agency: Behavioral organization from lizards to humans*. MIT Press.

Thornton, D. (2013). Implications of our developing understanding of risk and protective factors in the treatment of adult male sexual offenders. *International Journal of Behavioral Consultation and Therapy, 8*, 62–65.

Waldron, J. (2009). *Dignity, rank, and rights: The 2009 Tanner Lectures at UC Berkeley*. New York University of Law.

Ward, T. (2002). Good lives and the rehabilitation of sexual offenders: Promises and problems. *Aggression and Violent Behavior, 7*, 513–528.

Ward, T. (2010). The Good Lives model of offender rehabilitation: Basic assumptions, aetiological commitments, and practice implications. In F. McNeill, P. Raynor, & C. Trotter (Eds.), *Offender supervision: New directions in theory, research and practice*. Willan Publishing.

Ward, T. (2011). Human rights and dignity in offender rehabilitation. *Journal of Forensic Psychology Practice, 11*, 103–123.

Ward, T. (2013). Addressing the dual relationship problem in forensic and correctional practice. *Aggression and Violent Behavior, 18*, 92–100.

Ward, T. (2014). The explanation of sexual offending: From single factor theories to integrative pluralism. *Journal of Sexual Aggression, 20*, 130–141.

Ward, T. (2017). Prediction and agency: The role of protective factors in correctional rehabilitation and desistance. *Aggression and Violent Behavior, 32*, 19–28.

Ward, T., & Beech, A. R. (2015). Dynamic risk factors: A theoretical dead-end? *Psychology, Crime & Law, 21*, 100–113. https://doi.org/10.1080/1068316X.2014.917854

Ward, T., & Birgden, A. (2007). Human rights and correctional clinical practice. *Aggression and Violent Behavior, 12*, 628–643.

Ward, T., & Carter, E. (2019). The classification of offending and crime related problems: A functional perspective. *Psychology, Crime & Law, 25*, 542–560.

Ward, T., & Durrant, R. (2021). Practice frameworks in correctional psychology: Translating causal theories and normative assumptions into practice. *Aggression and Violent Behavior*. https://doi.org/10.1016/j.avb.2021.101612

Ward, T., & Durrant, R. (2022). Targets of explanation in forensic and correctional psychology: A black box model. *Aggression and Violent Behavior, 67*. https://doi.org/10.1016/j.avb.2022.101782

Ward, T., & Fisher, D. (2006). New ideas in the treatment of sexual offenders. In W. L. Marshall, Y. Fernandez, & L. Marshall (Eds.), *Sexual offender treatment: Issues and controversies* (pp. 143–158). John Wiley & Sons.

Ward, T., & Fortune, C. (2016). The role of dynamic risk factors in the explanation of offending. *Aggression and Violent Behavior, 29*, 79–88. https://doi.org/10.1016/j.avb.2016.06.007

Ward, T., Fox, A., & Garber, M. (2014). Restorative justice, offender rehabilitation, and desistance. *Restorative Justice: An International Journal, 2*, 24–42.

Ward, T., & Gannon, T. (2006). Rehabilitation, etiology, and self-regulation: The Good Lives Model of sexual offender treatment. *Aggression and Violent Behavior, 11*, 77–94.

Ward, T., Haig, D., & McDonald, M. (2022). Translating science into practice in clinical psychology: A reformulation of the evidence-based practice inquiry model. *Theory & Psychology, 32*, 401–422. https://doi.org/10.1177/09593543211059816

Ward, T., & Hudson, S. (2000). A self-regulation model of relapse prevention. In D. R. Lawes, S. M. Hudson, & T. Ward (Eds.), *Remaking relapse prevention with sex offenders: A sourcebook* (pp. 79–101). Sage.
Ward, T., & Laws, D. R. (2010). Desistance from sexual offending: Motivating change, enriching practice. *International Journal of Forensic Mental Health, 9*, 11–23.
Ward, T., & Marshall, W. L. (2004). Good lives, etiology and the rehabilitation of sex offenders: A bridging theory. *Journal of Sexual Aggression, 10*, 153–169.
Ward, T., & Maruna, S. (2007). *Rehabilitation: Beyond the risk paradigm*. Routledge.
Ward, T., & Stewart, C. A. (2003). Criminogenic needs and human needs: A theoretical model. *Psychology, Crime, & Law, 9*, 125–143.
Ward, T., Sullivan, J., & Durrant, R. (2024a). Epistemic disagreement in psychopathology research and practice: A procedural model. *Theory & Psychology, 34*, 484–507.
Ward, T., Vandevelde, S., & Wanzeele, W. (2024b). Theoretical innovations in the Good Lives Model. *Panopticon, 45*, 521–527.
Weaver, B., & McNeill, F. (2010). Travelling hopefully: Desistance research and probation practice. In F. Cowe, J. Deering, & J. Pakes (Eds.), *What else works? Creative work with offenders and other socially excluded people*. Cullompton, UK.
Willis, G., & Ward, T. (2024). Evidence for the Good Lives Model in supporting rehabilitation and desistance from offending. In L. A. Craig, L. Dixon, & T. A. Gannon (Eds.), *The Wiley handbook of what works in offender rehabilitation: An evidence-based approach to theory, assessment and treatment* (2nd ed.). Wiley-Blackwell.
Willis, G., Yates, P., Gannon, T., & Ward, T. (2013). How to integrate the good lives model into treatment programs for sexual offending: An introduction and overview. *Sexual Abuse: A Journal of Research and Treatment, 25*, 123–142.
Yates, P., Prescott, D., & Ward, T. (2010). *Applying the good lives model to sex offender treatment: A practical handbook for clinicians*. Safer Society Press.
Yates, P. M., & Prescott, D. S. (2011). *Building a better life: A good lives and self-regulation workbook*. Safer Society Press.
Yates, P. M., & Ward, T. (2008). Good lives, self-regulation, and risk management: An integrated model of sexual offender assessment and treatment. *Sexual Abuse in Australia and New Zealand: An Interdisciplinary Journal, 1*, 3–20.

Chapter 2
Incorporating Dynamic Risk Factors into GLM Case Formulations

2.1 Introduction

This chapter addresses the question of how to integrate dynamic risk factors (DRF) into a good lives model (GLM) informed assessment process and case formulation. A brief discussion of case formulation and its functions in clinical work will be followed by an examination of the way DRFs are typically used in forensic and correctional practice. In their standard form, they do not refer to causal factors and therefore are of limited value in explaining why clinical and offense-related problems occur and persist. Therefore, it is a mistake to see them as obstacles as they are not one thing; in fact, they are not any specific thing at all. Once you construct a GLM case formulation, DRFs simply disappear, and each can be broken down (deconstructed) into several different signal factors at different levels of analysis. The key task following a case formulation is the construction of a good lives plan in which the core competencies and external resources necessary for achieving prioritized goods are specified in detail.

2.2 What Is a Case Formulation and Why Is It Important?

Psychological assessment is the systematic collection of clinically relevant information through a variety of specific methods, including a clinical interview, administration of psychometric tests, behavioral observation, and a review of previous reports. There are several distinct assessment tasks, each requiring specific knowledge and skills, ranging from identifying problems to developing an explanatory model. More specifically, according to Ward et al. (2016) there are five major phases of clinical assessment: (a) establishing a focus of inquiry that spells out to the clinician exactly what it is they are hoping to achieve in the assessment process; (b)

T. Ward et al., *The Good Lives Model of Correctional Rehabilitation*,
Advances in Preventing and Treating Violence and Aggression,
https://doi.org/10.1007/978-3-031-95559-4_2

detecting a client's symptoms, signs, or problems (phenomena detection). This is a crucial step in assessment, as it is pointless to try developing an explanation of a client's offending until you have clearly pinpointed specific explanatory targets, such as persistent low mood, deviant sexual arousal, or social isolation. Focusing on offending behavior is too imprecise, as individuals who commit the same types of crime may have quite different problems; (c) inferring causes for each of these symptoms, signs, or problems (model generation); (d) developing an integrated case formulation of a specific person's range of problems (model development); and (e) evaluating the adequacy of the case formulation. Just how comprehensive and powerful is an explanation (model appraisal)? The methods used to collect assessment data are carefully chosen, and their reliability and validity established. The importance of data lies in the fact that they serve as evidence for clinical and offense-related phenomena under investigation.

It takes considerable knowledge and skill to develop a valid case formulation, and it is sometimes tempting for clinicians to base interventions on simple classification systems, such as offense categories, risk bands, or DRF (Ward & Carter, 2019). The challenges with using such treatment guidance strategies can be narrowed down to two main problems: (1) the categories are psychologically impoverished, containing very little useful clinical information; and (2) there is too much within category variability, that is, there are too many possible clinical presentations to be helpful for therapists (Ward & Carter, 2019). There is no real alternative to doing the hard work and striving to construct a rich model of a specific person's problems and their causes.

A good case formulation provides an understanding of what an individual's relevant offending and non-offending problems are, how they developed over time, what is causing them, and crucially, how the different causes interact with one another. The aim is to identify the etiological factors (i.e., initial exposure events such as loss, abuse, neglect, etc.) that resulted in the psychological vulnerabilities that lead to offending and non-offending related problems, and ideally, to specify the nature of the mechanisms constituting these vulnerabilities in some detail. For example, for an individual experiencing severe emotional neglect as a child could result in avoidant personality features and poor perspective-taking skills that culminate in consistent rejection by potential adult partners and subsequent violent behavior. The non-offending related problems linked to violent offending may be persistent loneliness, difficulty in dealing with social criticism, low mood, and so on.

2.3 The Standard Use of Dynamic Risk Factors in Forensic Practice

Both the concept of dynamic risk factors (DRFs) and the classification principles relating to that concept are at the center of contemporary forensic and correctional psychology (Bonta & Andrews, 2017; Mann et al., 2010; Ward & Durrant, 2021). The inclusion of DRFs to aid case formulations and inform treatment interventions has become standard clinical practice (Ward & Fortune, 2016), and it has been suggested that the specific DRFs most strongly associated with recidivism should be the primary focus of treatment (Mann et al., 2010). Individuals who have committed crimes are currently classified based on (a) the types of DRFs they are said to possess (e.g., intimacy deficit, self-regulation difficulties) and (b) the total number of DRFs that they have. For instance, Bonta and Andrews (2017) argue that an individual's level of risk is directly proportional to the number of risk factors present, and that the type and amount of DRFs present should facilitate the intensity and type of treatment prescribed.

Importantly, assigning DRFs to this role in understanding crime assumes that they can function as explanations of offending and constitute useful explanatory targets. Realistically, this is not the case (see Chap. 1 and below). While DRFs may display utility in the prediction of reoffending, they lack the specificity and theoretical coherence necessary to render them appropriate units of offender classification or causal factors. As argued in Chap. 1, the problems of poor specificity (i.e., DRFs refer to multiple possible causal factors), theoretical incoherence (i.e., they contain different types of concepts—causal, contextual, and "symptoms"), and their strongly normative nature (i.e., they are conceptually linked to offending behavior) mean that they are weak theoretical concepts (Ward, 2017; Ward & Beech, 2015; Ward & Fortune, 2016). This means each DRF is essentially a summary of variables that predict recidivism, and as such do not refer to any specific causal factors. One major difficulty is that because they are so closely associated with offending behavior, DRFs have little to offer clinicians in the way of clinical explanation and treatment guidance.

The argument that DRFs can be taken from the context of prediction to that of treatment has been made directly by Bonta and Andrews (2017) and Mann et al. (2010). The assumption seems to be that if DRFs are causes of offending and its related problems, then it makes sense to use them to formulate cases and guide treatment. There has also been a more cautious approach adopted by some researchers (Olver et al., 2022; Sturmey & McMurran, 2011; Sturmey et al., 2019; Thornton, 2013) who have pointed out that because DRFs are poorly conceptualized, they need to be developed in greater theoretical depth before they can be used clinically. However, despite this caution DRFs still play a prominent role in forensic case formulation chapters and papers, and there seems to be a reluctance to accept that they have very little to offer in both research and clinical explanatory contexts (Sturmey & McMurran, 2011).

2.3.1 Why Simply Reformulating DRF Does Not Work

There have been several attempts to overcome the conceptual problems evident in the standard Bonta and Andrews formulation of DRFs, none of which have been successful. Mann et al. (2010) and Thornton (2016) have provided two interesting reconceptualizations of DRFs.

Mann et al. (2010) identify a number of what they call psychologically meaningful risk factors, which may be prima facie causes of sexual offending and validated predictors of recidivism. They propose that to qualify as psychologically meaningful risk factors: (1) there should be plausible reasons for regarding the factor in question as a cause of sexual offending, and (2) strong evidence should exist that it actually predicts sexual offending. Mann and her colleagues suggest that another way to understand risk factors, instead of classifying them as static or dynamic, is by adopting the concept of psychologically meaningful risk factors. Such risk factors can be conceptualized as individual propensities to commit offenses, which may or may not manifest during any particular time period (p. 194). The list of empirically supported meaningful risk factors for child sexual abuse in their paper includes sexual preferences for children, emotional congruence with children, offense-supportive attitudes, and lack of adult intimate relationships.

Mann et al. (2010) assume that it is theoretically defensible to import the concept of dynamic risk factors from the prediction domain to the explanatory and practice domains without significantly reworking them. Relabeling dynamic risk factors as psychologically meaningful risk factors does not avoid the objection that they are, in part, normative concepts. This is because the criterion variable is offending behavior and, as such, is value-laden. Finally, the relationship between indicators of the various risk factors (e.g., score on scales, ratings by clinicians, etc.) and the latent construct (i.e., attributes, such as intimacy deficits), the dynamic risk factor, is unclear. How does the attribute cause the different values in score? How is it translated into response tendencies?

Thornton (2016) reworked the Mann et al. (2010) propensities model by placing greater emphasis on agency in the explanation and treatment of offending behavior, integrating the list of primary human goods from the good lives model (GLM) and drawing from Fishbein and Ajzen's Theory of reasoned action (2010). Thornton argues that an adequate account of DRFs needs to appeal to what people want from life and the translation of these desires into effective actions. He accepts that the GLM primary goods represent a reasonable list of the different types of desires found in human beings, which are expressed as goals in everyday life and longer-term plans. Over time, individuals develop schemas that contain representations of their environments and opportunities for securing specific goals arising from the more abstract PHGs. Specific action sequences (scripts and strategies) are gradually acquired and used in flexible ways toward the pursuit of valued goals. These scripts are like the GLM concepts of secondary goods and their associated good life plans. Thornton argues that when schemas and their associated goals and plans result in harmful outcomes, both to the person concerned and others, problems such as crime can occur. Inflexible schemas and plans can be caused by biological factors, problematic learning experiences, or shifting environmental demands. According to Thornton (2016), risk-related propensities "have their effect by increasing the psychological availability and attractiveness of antisocial behavioral options relative to the psychological availability and attractiveness of prosocial possibilities" (p. 143). In Thornton's model, DRFs are reflected in the inflexible operation of core schema, scripts, and strategies. Therapy according to this model crucially depends on realigning PHGs to prosocial goals by exposing individuals to peer and therapeutic pressure and by enhancing their self-regulation capacities.

Thornton's (2016) incorporation of agency and motivational concepts into an account of DRFs is a significant advance over the simple propensities model of Mann et al. (2010). It has similarities to the agency model of Heffernan and Ward (2023), and the enactivist model of criminal behavior developed in depth by Dent and Ward (2022). There are some weaknesses, however, that ultimately mean that it struggles to explain how maladaptive schemas relate to DRFs as they are formulated in risk prediction contexts. First, it is not clear how Thornton's model addresses the problems of poor specificity, incoherence, and the overreliance of DRF approaches on crime-related outcomes. Second, it does not account for the relationship between prioritized PHG and personal or practical identities and thus fails to unpack the importance of meaning or sense of purpose in therapeutically useful ways. Third, it overemphasizes the role of cognition and neglects that of emotions in accounting for the onset of crime and desistance from offending. According to the revised GLM (see Chap. 1), emotional processes are critical conduits between motivational systems and behavior in all domains of life. Finally, Thornton is unclear as to how clinicians could use DRFs when developing case formulations and planning treatment. Certainly, his model directs theoretical attention to psychological processes involved in all human behavior but exactly how do DRFs map onto these processes? Do they survive in some form? Do they genuinely refer to psychological and social factors, or are they simply useful "fictions"?

Ultimately, DRFs are psychometric not theoretical concepts and therefore are ill suited for explanatory purposes. More precisely, their hybrid nature makes them excellent predictive concepts but severely limits their value clinically. The fact that they do not pick out particular psychological or social factors would suggest there is no such thing in the world as a DRF. Instead, they are best viewed as summaries of heterogeneous variables that are associated with reoffending. There is often a confusion in the literature between DRFs as psychometric concepts and risk factors as specific causes or facets of the overarching DRFs in question. An example of this confusion is the way the DRF of emotional congruence with children is often used by clinicians. The DRF of emotional congruence contains multiple possible causal factors (specific risk factors), such as fear of adult relationships, poor intimacy skills, or perspective-taking problems. While each of these is a distinct risk factor, collectively they are part of the broader DRF of emotional congruence. When used clinically, it is the specific risk factor that should be referred to, not the overarching DRF of emotional congruence, which is simply a recidivism predictor. An example of this confusion is the Mann et al. (2010) list of psychologically meaningful causes, which are really DRFs, not risk factors in the narrower, causal sense. They are not the same thing, and treating them as such is likely to result in poorly directed therapy. A second conclusion is that it makes sense to build on the work of Thornton (2016) and start to think about motivational systems and their associated emotions and behavioral strategies in correctional and forensic treatment contexts. This means looking through individuals' offending behavior and inquiring into the core values and (often) implicit good life plans apparent in their day-to-day functioning, and to use this information to construct strength-based intervention plans. Understanding individuals' offending and non-offending problems through this lens means that critical questions are: What do people want? How are they going about realizing these desires and their associated goals? And why are they unsuccessful? From this perspective, it makes little sense to think of DRFs as discrete factors existing somewhere within the person and their environment. To put it a bit more colorfully, DRFs do not exist and therefore have little to offer clinicians when formulating cases and putting together treatment plans. However, they are helpful in *signaling* problem domains when used in conjunction with an explicit theory of motivation, emotion, and behavior.

2.4 How Case Formulation Should Proceed: Functional Domains

DRFs have been viewed by researchers as causes of criminal behavior, obstacles to the attainment of PHGs, propensities, and impairments in the conditions required for adaptive agency. Each of these positions has merit, but ultimately all fail to deal with the conceptual problems evident in formulations of DRFs. They all assume that DRFs in some way refer to specific causes, psychological problems, or contextual factors. Such mistaken assumptions are not uncommon in the literature (e.g., Heffernan et al., 2019; Ward & Fortune, 2016).

This section will lay the foundations for an alternative view: DRFs are predictive constructs, and the variables each one incorporates have very little in common other than some association with reoffending. While it makes sense to use them as initial estimates of reoffending and to monitor ongoing risk, the temptation to turn them into explanatory factors should be resisted. Rather, offending and non-offending problems can be effectively understood in terms of individuals' motivations, emotions, and strategies used to secure valued outcomes. A first step in developing a case formulation to guide treatment should be to identify the normative landscape within each person's life (e.g., what do they value, what are the expectations of the contexts within which they live, and so on). Once this has been done then the task is to describe the ways individuals go about achieving these outcomes in the contexts within which they live. This requires careful analysis of the specific motivational systems operating within the relevant contexts, their downstream emotions, and the plans used to realize the subsequent short- and long-term goals. DRFs can be useful to signal the salient motivational domains within which crime and its related problems are located, but that is all. The general motivational architecture employed in developing the good lives model is Del Giudice's motivational systems theory (2018, 2023).

2.4.1 Motivational Systems and Primary Human Goods

Research evidence from multiple disciplines suggests that human beings have several innate motivational systems and cognitive, behavioral, and physiological capacities designed to solve different adaptive problems (e.g., Aunger & Curtis, 2015; De Giudice, 2018, 2023; Gallagher, 2023; Kenrick et al., 2010; Tomasello, 2022). In proximal terms, these systems address a range of environmental challenges that individuals address using internal (e.g., skills, knowledge, capacities) and external resources (e.g., opportunities, social supports, education, work) acquired during their development and throughout their lives. The achievement of adaptive outcomes (i.e., reasonable levels of well-being) depends on having all needs met at least to a minimal degree (Alexandrova, 2017; Ward & Maruna, 2007). De Giudice (2018, p.37) expresses this pluralistic conception of human motivation and its relationship to behavior well:

> In sum, motivational systems set the goals of behavior and monitor causes of success and failure in the pursuit of those goals. Motivational systems affect behavior indirectly by triggering emotions, which in turn coordinate adaptive suites of physiological, cognitive, and behavioral responses.

The life history theory approach of Del Giudice (2018, p.40–45) to the classification and explanation of psychopathology is helpful in identifying a plausible list of motivational systems causing offending behavior and its associated problems. According to Del Giudice (2018), the evolutionary, neuroscience, and psychological evidence points to the existence of several motivational systems adaptations that have evolved because of their contribution to human beings' inclusive fitness. These systems frequently act in conjunction with one another, because (a) people might be pursuing multiple goals at the same time, and/or (b) several systems may be contributing to the achievement of a single outcome (e.g., a romantic relationship, which arguably taps into care giving, mating, and attachment systems). The following includes some minor modifications to Del Giudice's list of motivational systems and some merged to simplify the discussion (Del Giudice, 2018). Given the constraints of this chapter, only a brief description of each system is included, along with the primary human goods that appear to be linked to each one (see Ward & Carter, 2019 for a fuller discussion).

The *bodily regulation system* is responsible for motivating individuals to attend to their physical needs such as the need for warmth, fluids, nutrition, sleep, sex, and regulated temperature (GLM primary human good of life). The function of the *aggression motivational system* is to respond to threats of harm to oneself or loved ones by some kind of aggressive action and the proactive pursuit of dominance (GLM primary human goods of life, agency, relationships, and inner peace). The *fear and security motivational systems* function to enable people to avoid or escape from immediate threats to their safety or detect and prevent possible threats from occurring in the future. The *motivational system of disgust* serves to make sure people avoid contact with material that might contain pathogens, such as waste products, rotting food, diseased individuals, and moral or social pollution in order to prevent contamination (GLM primary human goods of relationships, community, life). Moral or social disgust can manifest as a strong aversion to people with different sexual orientations or from minority ethnic groups and in some circumstances cause individuals to physically harm members from despised groups. The *status motivational system* motivates people to compete for high social status and act in ways that maintain their position once they have achieved the desired level of social recognition (GLM primary human goods of relationships, community, agency). The *mating system and pair bonding systems* are concerned with the initial discovery, attraction, and selection of sexual partners and the establishment of long-term adult sexual or romantic relationships (GLM primary human goods of relationships, pleasure, inner peace). The *attachment system and caregiving systems* enable individuals to provide, acquire, or obtain care and support within a close relationship, whether a parent, friend, or romantic partner. The availability of a caring, loving person provides emotional support to individuals when they need it (GLM primary human goods of relationships, agency, community). The *affiliation motivational system* encourages people to seek out relationships with non-family members and to establish and maintain strong relationships with members of their social group (GLM primary human goods of community, relationships). The r*eciprocity and acquisition systems* facilitate fair trade and interactions between people, to monitor compliance to shared norms, and to detect and punish cheaters, while the acquisition system motivates persons to acquire and protect their resources (GLM primary human goods of work, agency, and community). The *play motivational system* motivates individuals to acquire and develop physical, social, and cognitive skills in non-threatening contexts (GLM primary human goods of play, relationships). The mastery of these competencies also provides them with the opportunity to display to others their level of skill, and in this respect, signals prowess and social attractiveness. The *curiosity motivational system* prompts people to acquire knowledge about the way the world works and to find out why people act as they do (GLM primary human goods of knowledge, creativity, relationships, spirituality). From a social cognition perspective, the knowledge gained helps social groups to coalesce and individuals to form enduring and loving relationships.

A few things are worth commenting on with respect to the relationship between the GLM and motivational systems. First, while the above motivational systems prompt individuals to seek certain goals, they require specific sets of cognitive, emotional, behavioral, and physiological capacities if they are to achieve the desired outcomes. Without these internal and external capacities, it is unlikely that an individual will successfully achieve the goals in a fulfilling and adaptive manner. The actual suite of internal and external resources necessary to obtain goals, such as romantic relationships or just outcomes, depends on the environments/contexts in which individuals live and the resources or constraints they contain. Furthermore, the specific plans used to pursue goals specified by each system require higher level cognitive abilities, and as such, are likely to be linked to the primary human good of agency. Dysfunctions in the various motivational systems and/or impairments in the capacities required to attain the relevant goals are associated with dynamic risk factors. Second, in each of these motivational systems, the range of problems experienced by people are likely to extend beyond their offending behavior and be visible in their day-to-day lives in multiple ways. This prompts researchers and practitioners to look at the broader picture and regard offenses as simply one aspect or symptom of broader clusters of difficulties, loosely organized by motivational systems. From a GLM perspective, asking "What task(s) is the person attempting to complete in what specific environment?" is more likely to provide a valid way of identifying the challenges faced by people who commit crimes. Third, sometimes the outcomes for individuals may be beneficial in the specific contexts in which they live and should not be regarded as necessarily indicating psychological deficits, even if they are illegal. This entails that it would be a waste of valuable resources offering such individuals therapy. Fourth, emotions play a crucial role in creating prioritized goals(values) and good life plans, and points to the clinical importance of accessing the emotions underlying values in intervention work.

De Guidice's model of motivational systems provides a strong research basis for the GLM list of primary human goods, which are surface-level descriptions of the kind of goals people seek in their day-to-day lives. PHGs are relatively superficial descriptions, in part, because they have been derived by conceptual analysis and statistical methods like factor analysis, which simply derives categories based on correlations. The model of motivational systems, on the other hand, goes further to explain why human beings are strongly motivated to seek certain outcomes (they are adaptations), why they arise in response to salient environmental and internal cues, and how they result in the formation of good life plans (via emotion and its downstream coordination of responses and behavior). In effect, PHGs can be best understood as clinical glosses on motivational systems and more user-friendly for clinical work with clients who have offended.

2.4.2 *Motivational Systems and Dynamic Risk Factors*

On analysis, DRFs disappear as distinct causal factors and manifest in diverse types of problems across agent-action-context sequences, at different levels of analysis. Practitioners should resist any temptation to regard them (1) as causal factors in their standard formulation (Bonta & Andrews, 2017; Mann et al., 2010) or (2) causes once deconstructed into their causal components. This is because they are so strongly linked to offending behavior that individuals' major life concerns and offense-related problems can be overlooked and treatment skewed toward the identification and management of risk factors. A consequence of this gravitational trap is a narrowness of treatment and difficulty engaging individuals in the process of developing alternative good life plans. The relatively modest effectiveness of risk-management approaches, such as the RNR (Fazel et al., 2024) and parallel research from psychotherapy points to the necessity of building intervention plans around a person's core values and the therapeutic relationships (Wampold, 2019). Viewing individuals through a risk lens can create a disconnect between therapist and client, which can result in ongoing therapeutic ruptures that may be difficult to repair

(Gannon & Ward, 2014). In a nutshell, DRFs are best used as signaling devices or indicators of problems within well-being-related domains, such as relationships or emotional competence. They should not be used as causal factors within case formulations.

The following steps are helpful when using DRFs in clinical assessment:

1. *The initial starting point* in assessment is identifying the PHG(s) associated with motivational systems and the psychological processes evident in a person's life at the time of their offending. This can be done using the GLM tools reviewed in Chap. 3, including the mapping table.
2. DRFs can serve as additional signaling systems that point to the relevant motivational systems and associated PHGs and life plans with their values in play (van den Berg et al., 2022). For example, emotional congruence with children could pick up difficulties with intimacy and relationships, while negative emotionality/hostility may suggest agency and status seeking problems. The key issue is that each DRF has multiple components and can, at best, only provide tentative evidence for judgments concerning what motivational systems and PHGs are salient for any given individual.
3. Once the motivational systems along with the emotions and goals caused by them are identified, the next step is to describe the psychological and contextual components constituting the scripts and good life plans active within a person's life at the time of their offending.
4. The consequences of these active motivational systems and consequent emotions should be identified, and their relationships to the problems associated with an individual's offending and in their lives overall should be noted. This is a descriptive task resulting in a list of clinical phenomena experienced by the individual being assessed.
5. At this point, DRFs no longer have a useful role, and the process of developing a case formulation should proceed. A GLM case formulation seeks to explain offending and non-offending clinical phenomena within the context of the individual and his/her life. It includes stipulating the function/purpose of offending for the individual and, crucially, detecting the individual's prioritized PHGs and the relationship to their practical identity. This involves arriving at a careful description of a maladaptive life plan and its constituent obstacles, namely, problems with means, capacity, scope, and conflict.
6. A good lives intervention plan based on the identification of core motivational systems, goals, and plans should be constructed and used to guide therapy. This will have risk-reducing and well-being enhancing elements (see Chap. 4). For example, devising alternative prosocial ways of establishing social status, or affiliative networks.

2.5 Conclusion

DRFs are the children of risk prediction. They were originally identified to help practitioners assess risk of recidivism and set treatment targets likely to reduce reoffending. Unfortunately, this dual role is seriously undermined by their poor specificity, lack of coherence, and weak explanatory power. It is tempting to accept the dual-purpose conceptualization of DRFs as recidivism predictors and as causes of offending and non-offending problems. It is tempting because it seems to offer an elegant and parsimonious approach to assessment and treatment planning. However, this temptation should be resisted because it is based on the mistaken assumption that DRFs can be translated into causal factors in a relatively simple way. Rather, DRFs are summaries of variables associated with offending, which on their own do not reveal much about why people act in harmful ways toward other people or experience psychological and social problems. Quite simply, they are not causal concepts. A more worthwhile approach is to view them as signaling devices that highlight important themes in people's lives (PHGs) around the time they offended. As such, they can inform case formulation and treatment planning. Interestingly, the conceptual problems of poor specificity, incoherence, grain, and their value-laden nature actually make DRFs perfect signaling devices because breadth of coverage increases their signaling power. Therefore, they have a theoretical virtue in this context rather than being problematic when used to construct causal explanations.

References

Alexandrova, A. (2017). *A philosophy for the science of well-being*. Oxford University Press.

Aunger, R., & Curtis, V. (2015). *Gaining control: How human behaviour evolved*. Oxford University Press. https://doi.org/10.1176/appi.books.9780890425596

Bonta, J., & Andrews, D. A. (2017). *The psychology of criminal conduct* (6th ed.). Routledge.

Del Giudice, M. (2018). *Evolutionary psychopathology: A unified approach*. Oxford University Press.

Del Giudice, M. (2023). A general motivational architecture of human and animal personality. *Neuroscience and Biobehavioral Reviews, 144*. https://doi.org/10.1016/j.neubiorev.2022.104967

Dent, H., & Ward, T. (2022). Emotion and correctional practice: Theoretical foundations of an enactive practice framework. *Aggression and Violent Behavior, 63*. https://doi.org/10.1016/j.avb.2021.101672

Fazel, S., Hurton, C., Burghart, M., Delisi, M., & Yu, R. (2024). An updated evidence synthesis on the Risk-Need-Responsivity (RNR) model: Umbrella review and commentary. *Journal of Criminal Justice, 92*. https://doi.org/10.1016/j.jcrimjus.2024.102197

Fishbein, M., & Ajzen, I. (2010). *Predicting and changing behavior: The reasoned action approach*. Psychology Press (Taylor & Francis).

Gallagher, S. (2023). *Embodied and enactive approaches to cognition*. Cambridge University Press.

Gannon, T., & Ward, T. (2014). Where has all the psychology gone? A critical review of evidence-based psychological practice in correctional settings. *Aggression and Violent Behavior, 19*, 435–436.

Heffernan, R., & Ward, T. (2023). Offering the possibility of better lives: A strength based approach to social reintegration. In F. Coppola & A. Murtufi (Eds.), *Social rehabilitation and punishment: Legal, empirical, and penological perspectives*. Routledge.

Heffernan, R., Wegerhoff, D., & Ward, T. (2019). Dynamic risk factors: Conceptualization, measurement, and evidence. *Aggression and Violent Behavior, 48*, 6–16.

Kenrick, D. T., Griskevicius, V., Neuberg, S. L., & Schaller, M. (2010). Renovating the pyramid of needs: Contemporary extensions: built upon ancient foundations. *Perspectives on Psychological Science, 5*, 292–314. https://doi.org/10.1177/1745691610369469

Mann, R. E., Hanson, R. K., & Thornton, D. (2010). Assessing risk for sexual recidivism: Some proposals on the nature of psychologically meaningful risk factors. *Sexual Abuse: A Journal of Research and Treatment, 22*, 191–217. https://doi.org/10.1177/1079063210366039

Olver, M. E., Thornton, D., & Beggs Christofferson, S. M. (2022). Understanding the latent structure of dynamic risk: Seeking empirical constraints on theory development using the VRS-SO and the theory of dynamic risk. *Sexual Abuse, 34*, 227–254. https://doi.org/10.1177/10790632211 10028

Sturmey, P., & McMurran, M. (Eds.). (2011). *Forensic case formulation*. Wiley.

Sturmey, P., McMurran, M., & Daffern, M. (2019). In D. L. L. Polaschek, A. Day, & C. R. Hollin (Eds.), *The Wiley international handbook for correctional psychology* (pp. 476–487).

Thornton, D. (2013). Implications of our developing understanding of risk and protective factors in the treatment of adult male sexual offenders. *International Journal of Behavioral Consultation and Therapy, 8*, 62–65.

Thornton, D. (2016). Developing a theory of dynamic risk. *Psychology, Crime, & Law, 22*, 138–150.

Tomasello, M. (2022). *The evolution of agency: Behavioral organization from lizards to humans*. MIT Press.

van den Berg, J. W., et al. (2022). Dynamic risk factors in adult men who committed sexual offenses: Replication and comparison of networks found in two independent samples. *Psychology of Violence, 2*, 424–437. https://doi.org/10.1037/vio0000445.supp

Wampold, B. E. (2019). *The basics of psychotherapy: An introduction to theory and practice* (2nd ed.). American Psychological Association.

Ward, T. (2017). Prediction and agency: The role of protective factors in correctional rehabilitation and desistance. *Aggression and Violent Behavior, 32*, 19–28.

Ward, T., & Beech, A. R. (2015). Dynamic risk factors: A theoretical dead-end? *Psychology, Crime & Law, 21*, 100–113. https://doi.org/10.1080/1068316X.2014.917854

Ward, T., Clack, S., & Haig, B. (2016). The Abductive theory of method: Scientific inquiry and clinical practice. *Behaviour Change, 33*, 212–231.

Ward, T., & Carter, E. (2019). The classification of offending and crime related problems: A functional perspective. *Psychology, Crime & Law, 25*, 542–560.

Ward, T., & Fortune, C. (2016). The role of dynamic risk factors in the explanation of offending. *Aggression and Violent Behavior, 29*, 79–88. https://doi.org/10.1016/j.avb.2016.06.007

Ward, T., & Maruna, S. (2007). *Rehabilitation: Beyond the risk paradigm*. Routledge.

Ward, T., & Durrant, R. (2021). Practice frameworks in correctional psychology: Translating causal theories and normative assumptions into practice. *Aggression and Violent Behavior, 58*. https://doi.org/10.1016/j.avb.2021.101612

Chapter 3
Assessment Framework and Issues

3.1 Introduction

The Good Lives Model (GLM) provides an overarching framework for forensic/correctional rehabilitation, informing all stages of intervention. It is intended to help facilitate client engagement from the very first interaction; however, offending treatment programs that purport to use the GLM often omit or minimally implement the GLM into preprogram clinical assessments (Prescott & Willis, 2021; Willis et al., 2014). Intake and assessment practices generally focus primarily or exclusively on Risk, Need, and Responsivity (RNR; Bonta & Andrews, 2017) considerations, with the GLM informing specific program content and/or the general delivery of offense-focused treatment. That is, even in programs advocating a GLM approach, assessment practices tend to focus on identification of dynamic risk factors (DRFs)/criminogenic needs, and an exploration of potential responsivity barriers to engaging in offense-focused treatment. A mismatch between risk-oriented assessment and strengths-based treatment is not surprising considering correctional psychology's emphasis on clinician-rated risk assessment tools, which help triage clients for appropriate levels of intervention intensity. Inconsistent with a GLM approach, however, DRFs identified by clinician-rated tools are often transcribed directly into therapy plans. Such a process presents two dilemmas: First, identifying therapy goals through a risk lens is at odds with the strengths-based approach central to the GLM. Second, DRFs share a correlational relationship with reoffending; they do not pinpoint sources of risk requiring intervention (Heffernan et al., 2019; Ward, 2016). They should be used as signaling devices not as causal concepts and subsequent treatment targets (see Chaps. 1 and 2). This chapter will describe how to implement the GLM in pretreatment clinical assessments alongside RNR considerations. Further discussion will illustrate how the structured assessment of protective factors within the broader GLM practice framework can support an assessment process aligned with RNR considerations that is strengths-based, capitalizing on opportunities to engage clients at the earliest

T. Ward et al., *The Good Lives Model of Correctional Rehabilitation*,
Advances in Preventing and Treating Violence and Aggression,
https://doi.org/10.1007/978-3-031-95559-4_3

opportunity. When it is clear from the outset that clinicians are invested in getting to know clients beyond their offending and risk factors, clients may be more invested in the assessment process.

3.2 A GLM-Grounded Assessment Framework

A comprehensive assessment is fundamental to informing therapy goals aligned with the GLM's dual aims of risk reduction alongside supporting clients to live meaningful, satisfying lives. The overall aim of the clinical assessment is to gather sufficiently detailed information to develop a working case formulation of a client's offending behavior and associated obstacles encountered in seeking out primary human goods (PHGs) in meaningful, adaptive ways. The case formulation—not simply a list of DRFs—then informs therapy goals. As stated in Chap. 2, DRFs need to be broken down into their associated components to be of any clinical use in case formulation. Although this chapter focuses on the pretreatment assessment phase, it is important to emphasize that the assessment process is necessarily ongoing as the therapeutic relationship strengthens and clients become more acquainted with the therapeutic process. Accordingly, the case formulation should be updated as more information is shared. This chapter focuses on pertinent GLM considerations within clinical assessment. We refer readers to Ward et al. (2017) for a comprehensive clinical assessment framework.

Using the GLM, a client's implicit Good Life Plan (GLP) at relevant life stages provides an overarching template for assessment. That is, the focus of assessment is on understanding the client's GLPs, including PHGs prioritized, associated means used to attain PHGs (i.e., secondary goods), and strengths and obstacles experienced in pursuing their GLPs. Consistent with the GLM's emphasis on strengthening client agency, the sequencing of assessment tasks can be flexible and must be negotiated with the client. Some clients may present with high levels of anxiety and volunteer very little about themselves, in which case validating their anxiety and offering the least threatening starting place (e.g., an initial focus on the client's current GLP) can be helpful. Other clients may have waited a long time to speak with a clinician and present as eager to talk about their offending and its precipitants, in which case an initial focus on the client's GLP at the time of offending may be helpful. Wherever the starting place, assessment ultimately aims to uncover (i.e., make explicit) the client's GLP(s) during periods of offending and the client's current GLP.[1]

Clinicians explore GLPs initially through open-ended questions paired with a warm, inviting therapeutic approach where they show genuine interest in the client's current and past lived experiences. Next, they explore the full range of PHGs,

[1] It is important to distinguish between GLP associated with offending and offending-related problems from a therapeutic GLP that is derived from a comprehensive assessment process, which informs intervention and the desistance process.

including strengths and obstacles to goods attainment. Several tools/resources have been developed to help clinicians gather and integrate relevant information with different clients and in different contexts, including forensic mental health (Barnao, 2013), case management (Purvis et al., 2011, 2013), with adults who have sexually offended (Yates et al., 2009, 2010), and with young people who have sexually offended (Print, 2013). This chapter offers examples of tools which readers may wish to use and/or adapt to suit their setting and/or client group. As a practice framework, the GLM is not prescriptive; it allows a flexible approach to assessment that is responsive to the client's context, presenting concerns, and responsivity considerations.

3.2.1 Exploring the GLP: Identifying Primary Human Goods

Interview assessment starts with a series of broad, open-ended questions to map out the client's current and past priorities and commitments. An exploratory interview process follows, with the explicit aim of identifying underlying PHGs. This process is akin to peeling back layers of an onion, with the outermost layers representing secondary goods and the inner layers representing PHGs. The following questions might support initial examination of the client's current GLP: "I'm interested in getting to know you, and what's important in your life. Is there some place you might like to start?" "What do you value most in your life?" "What are you longing for in your life?" "What's missing from your life that you wish was there?" "What are the most important things for you to achieve in your life?" A semi-structured interview guide based on the interview schedule provided in Barnao (2013) offers additional/complementary questions, and is appended to this chapter (see Appendix A). When working with clients with cognitive impairments, the process of identifying PHGs might be aided by the use of visual materials (e.g., picture cards, magazines) or exploring different fictional characters the client admires and why.

It is important that identifying prioritized PHGs follows a process of detection achieved through reflective listening, paraphrasing, and summarizing—and not through presenting clients with a written list of PHGs and asking them to identify their relative importance. PHGs are relatively abstract concepts, and when asked about their core commitments and what matters most in their lives, clients will often volunteer secondary goods—what they do/did in relation to PHGs. The following questions might help to identify the relevant underlying PHGs:

> What does (*secondary good*) mean to you? And if you had that, then what would you have in your life? And if you had that, then what would you have in your life? *(continue until an underlying PHG/s is identified)*. What would that give you, provide for you, mean to you?

As underlying PHGs are identified, the therapist can validate the client's pursuit of valued goods, emphasizing that the client has the same rights to seek and attain them as any other person. Exploration of PHGs provides opportunities to legitimize client hopes and aspirations and to communicate to the client their inherent value as a fellow human being, worthy of experiences that bring them fulfillment and meaning in life. Additionally, the exploration of PHGs can help facilitate therapeutic self-disclosure supportive of rapport building (e.g., "I get that, I too desire close relationships in my life").

As clients share information relevant to their current GLP, the clinician might ask permission to explore different areas in more detail. Here, the clinician aims to identify secondary goods or means used to secure the range of PHGs, along with strengths and obstacles to goods attainment. Depending on the client's responses to early questions, the following questions might support deeper exploration:

> You've highlighted the importance of (*identify emerging PHGs*) in your life. If it's okay with you, can we explore these areas some more?
>
> Relationships are clearly important to you. Tell me about your relationships, who are the important people in your life?

Exploring the client's GLP(s) during period(s) of offending follows a similar approach to exploring the client's current GLP. Using open-ended questions and a nonjudgmental stance the clinician might invite the client to share what their life looked like, including their life priorities and concerns, in the lead up to their offending. The clinician might ask "What were you hoping to achieve?" and/or "What were you looking for/longing for?" From here, they can explore the client's offending through a series of increasingly detailed questions that focus not on explicit details of the offense(s), but on the function of offending behavior with respect to the pursuit of good life goals (i.e., means to attain PHGs). In the event clients disagree with or deny official reports of offending, the clinician can explore what was happening in the lead up to an accusation of offending behavior (Wanzeele & Seys, 2023). The focus should be on developing a working understanding of the PHGs implicated in the offense process and their life more generally at the time of offending. Some PHGs may have been sought directly through offending behavior; for example, sexual offending may relate to the problematic pursuit of relatedness, inner peace, agency and/or states of happiness and pleasure. Residential burglary often relates to the problematic pursuit of life (Taylor, 2017), whereas violence may relate to agency, and substance use to inner peace and/or states of happiness and pleasure. The clinician can validate underlying PHGs as they are identified, without condoning the offending behavior. Other times, offending relates indirectly to the pursuit of PHGs. In the absence of an explicit intention to offend, problems can arise in the pursuit of PHGs, which ultimately culminate in a criminal offense (i.e., there is cascade effect—see Chap. 1). For example, losing a job/contract and associated financial stress (PHG: life) may lead to stressors within an intimate partner relationship (PHG: relatedness), with combined stressors eventually exhausting an individual's coping capacity, impacting on PHGs of inner peace and states of happiness and pleasure. Offending (e.g., sexual offending, drug-related offending) may reflect a maladaptive attempt to regain a sense of inner peace and/or states of happiness and pleasure. Appendix B provides a template which can be used to support assessment of primary goods around the time of offending. Exploring goods implicated in offending continues through early stages of therapy as clients develop their own understanding of their offense process (see Chap. 4—intervention framework). A comprehensive understanding of PHGs implicated in offending is fundamental to informing priorities for therapy and risk management.

3.2.2 *Exploring the GLP: Identifying Obstacles to Goods Attainment*

Knowledge-related assumptions of the GLM emphasize that offending and life problems relate to obstacles implementing a Good Life Plan (GLP). The GLM defines four kinds of obstacles: problematic *means,* where the instrumental or secondary goods used in pursuit of PHGs are maladaptive and/or harmful; narrow *scope*, where an individual focuses narrowly on selected PHG(s) and neglects other prioritized goods; *conflict* or a lack of coherence in means used to attain different PHGs, or in the prioritization of PHGs; and finally, problems with *capacity* within the client (internal capacity) and/or in their environment (external capacity) to seek out primary goods in adaptive, meaningful ways. Obstacles can be explored initially through open-ended questions such as "What has gotten in the way of you living the life you want for yourself?" or "What challenges have you faced?" Clinicians can acknowledge that we all experience challenges from time to time, and some challenges are commonly associated with different types of offending behavior and life problems. For example, the clinician might reflect "some people with a history of sexual offending against children describe a sense of closeness to children/young people that they may have struggled to experience with adults. I'm interested in your experiences of emotional closeness." In this example, a traditionally defined risk factor (emotional connection to children) is reframed as a maladaptive secondary good. Obstacles are explored in relation to all PHGs prioritized by the client, and those implicated in their offending. Problems with *scope* and *conflict* are isolated through evaluation of an individual's entire lifestyle to identify PHGs that may be important but not attained (indicative of problems with scope) and PHGs (or secondary goods) that compete with each other (indicative of conflict). As they explore obstacles, clients may volunteer information relevant to mental health difficulties and other possible *responsivity* considerations. Accordingly, during discussions of obstacles to implementing GLPs, clinicians can collect information relevant to completing mental health screens. It is important for clinicians to take a trauma-informed approach to understanding obstacles and recognize that problems with capacity often reflect what has happened to clients over the course of their lives. Often, early adversities will have resulted in maladaptive behaviors and restricted opportunities to seek out PHGs in prosocial ways (see Levenson & Willis, 2019; Levenson et al., 2017). Problems with internal capacity can also relate to congenital conditions, including sensory impairments and intellectual disabilities. Problems with external capacity may include a lack of resources or opportunities to seek out PHGs. Historical trauma holds relevance to external capacity, and it is important that the clinician actively recognizes inequities experienced by indigenous and ethnic minority groups in their access to healthcare, employment, and other adaptive means for securing PHGs. Likewise, it is important that clinicians recognize inequities experienced by other marginalized groups, including sexual and gender minorities, in their access to PHGs. Barnao (2013) developed an interview guide and GLM mapping table to support exploration of strengths and obstacles to goods attainment and to integrate relevant information. Adapted versions of each are provided in Appendix B and C, respectively.

3.3 Risk Assessment Within the GLM Practice Framework

As we have illustrated in earlier chapters, the GLM accommodates RNR principles. Accordingly, an assessment of recidivism risk (although not required for GLM-based intervention) can be achieved within the GLM's overarching strengths-based framework. An important key function of risk assessment within a broader GLM framework is to help inform allocation of correctional resources and not infer treatment needs. Per the risk principle, clients assessed with an above average risk for reoffending will require a greater intensity of intervention and supervision than clients assessed in lower risk categories. Client records can provide information required to score static risk instruments, which include historical risk indicators like the number of prior convictions. Information required to score dynamic risk instruments, comprising such psychological and social risk indicators as peer associations and self-regulation capacity, can be collected as part of the broader exploration of problems with capacity implementing a GLP (also see Chap. 2). Importantly, these data are collected through a strengths-based lens. To reiterate from Chap. 1, within the GLM, DRFs are conceptualized as proxies for impairments in an individual's capacities to seek out PHGs in adaptive ways (i.e., as signaling devices). They can function as signals or crude indicators to clusters of capacity, conflict, means, and scope problems. They can point to the motivational systems, related PHG(s), and secondary goods associated with offending- and nonoffending-related problems. Readers familiar with commonly used dynamic risk assessment tools will appreciate that their accompanying interview protocols (and focus on problems, deficits, and risk) often run contrary to the GLM's emphasis on strengthening capacity to live a better life. Consideration of *protective factors*, on the other hand, aligns well with such a focus. Protective factors represent proxies for strengths in an individual's capacity to implement a prosocial GLP. An exploration of clients' existing strengths (important to maintain and to cultivate) and those in need of developing fits better within the strengths-based framework of the GLM than an exploration of risk factors that need to be reduced or managed.

Risk assessments inform many decisions in the criminal justice system, and there is often an expectation that multiple risk tools are scored. Regardless of which tools are used (clinicians may have limited choices), switching from a focus on assessing risk factors to a focus on assessing protective factors supports a risk assessment process that is strengths-based. Preliminary work by Willis et al. (2024) demonstrated that an assessment of protective factors using the Structured Assessment of PROtective Factors against Sexual Offending (SAPROF-SO; Willis et al., 2022) identified the same risk proxies as commonly used dynamic risk assessment tools, namely, the Stable-2007 (Fernandez et al., 2014; Hanson et al., 2007) and Violence Risk Scale—Sexual Offense version (Wong et al., 2003–2017). Accordingly, at least in the context of sexual recidivism risk assessment, an assessment of protective factors can provide data relevant to scoring dynamic risk tools.

Alongside informing an overall assessment of relative risk and inferring therapy foci, contemporary dynamic risk assessment instruments are often used to assess pre/post treatment change. For example, the VRS-SO includes change ratings for each DRF identified as a treatment need (although according to the GLM, they are not the focus of interventions but rather indicators of problem clusters). Notwithstanding the problems previously discussed with structuring intervention plans around DRFs (see Chap. 2), demands of justice system processes (e.g., parole board hearings) require clinicians to comment on how much clients have made change that can be linked (even if just statistically) with a reduced likelihood of reoffending. Communicating change through a protective factors lens aligns more closely with the GLM's focus on building capacity than communicating change through a focus on DRFs. Additionally, protective factor instruments, including the SAPROF (de Vogel et al., 2012) and SAPROF-SO, consider a broader range of variables than dynamic risk instruments, including those associated with desistance from offending that are not captured by dynamic risk tools. For example, the SAPROF-SO *Goal-directed living* item considers the presence of personally meaningful approach-oriented goals and the extent to which those goals motivate prosocial behavior. In other words, *Goal-directed living* is consistent with the GLM's focus on supporting individuals to actively work toward good life goals. Therapy progress associated with working toward good life goals might be missed when an assessment of treatment change relies on dynamic risk assessment instruments alone.

It is important to emphasize that the use of protective factor instruments to help infer therapy goals, although they may be strengths-based, suffer from the same dilemmas as using dynamic risk instruments to infer therapy goals. That is, protective factors reflect measurable, often composite constructs correlated with an absence of reoffending and are not necessarily causally related with desistance from crime (Ward, 2017). In other words, they lack explanatory depth and by extension, may flag but not necessarily pinpoint relevant therapy foci; they signal relevant strengths. Protective factor instruments can offer a useful check that risk-relevant propensities are accounted for in the therapy plan; however, it is the case formulation that ultimately informs specific therapy goals. Individualized case formulations (and not lists of DRFs or protective factors) are central to effective practice in forensic and clinical psychology and can help identify sources of risk for an individual client (Gannon & Ward, 2014; Vess et al., 2008). To illustrate, a lack of emotional connections with adults (the presence of which is a protective factor in the SAPROF-SO) might originate in several different underlying causal processes each signaling differing approaches to intervention. For example, longstanding social anxiety may have created a barrier to developing friendships and relationships with same-aged peers, and children may have been viewed as less threatening. Alternatively, a lack of emotional connections to adults may reside in entrenched maladaptive schemas about the trustworthiness of others. In other cases, schizoid personality traits and/or autism spectrum disorder might underlie poorly developed emotional connections to others. The protective factor is therefore best seen as a flag or proxy for a therapy goal, and the underlying process responsible for that proxy—identified via the case formulation—will help pinpoint relevant therapy goals and their relative importance in terms of addressing an individual's risk and supporting their future pursuit of good life goals.

3.4 From Assessment to Intervention/Therapy Planning

As we have discussed, a client's good life plan (GLP) at relevant life stages (i.e., at the time(s) of offending and at assessment) provides an overarching template for assessment. Likewise, the GLP provides a template for a rehabilitation plan, which sets out a plan for overcoming obstacles in pursuit of PHGs. Such a plan will likely include specific psychological therapy components to support strengthening internal capacity alongside recreational, vocational, and/or social components to support strengthening external capacity. It helps to structure the intervention plan around PHGs that are important to the client currently along with those goods implicated in offending. Several available tools and templates can support developing a cohesive rehabilitation plan (e.g., Barnao, 2013), most of which structure the intervention plan around how the client will fulfill each of the GLM's PHGs. An alternative approach is to organize the intervention plan around good life goals (future-oriented secondary goods), especially when clients can already articulate several adaptive, meaningful, and realistic goals. It is not uncommon for specific good life goals to map onto (i.e., provide a source of) multiple PHGs, and organizing the intervention plan around good life goals can therefore support generation of an individualized and coherent intervention plan. Further, organizing the plan around good life goals may help promote client agency as the plan's grounding is in their goals for a better life, rather than the GLM's emphasis on 11 PHGs. As emphasized in Chap. 1, we expect most clients will seek out most PHGs at least to some degree. However, selected PHGs may feature minimally in some clients' conceptualizations of a good life, and it is not our intent to suggest a client's GLP must account for every PHG. Appendix D provides a template for a rehabilitation plan structured around PHGs and we will illustrate an alternative template organized around good life goals with a case example in the next section. Regardless of the structure of the rehabilitation plan, the important things are that the client's good life goals and relevant strengths in need of development (i.e., internal and external capacity needs) are clearly articulated and that the plan demonstrates coherence and sufficient scope.

To reiterate, good life goals represent meaningful secondary/instrumental goods that will (or in the case of existing strengths, do) provide sources of PHG(s). As good life goals are identified, the therapist explores with the client what capacities require development for the good life goals to be realized (i.e., strengths in need of development to implement a good life plan). The initial case formulation provides a foundation from which to identify capacities in need of development. For example, in the context of poorly developed emotion regulation capacity that perpetuates violence and/or verbal aggression in the context of interpersonal conflict, supporting the client to develop adaptive emotion regulation skills can be an important therapy component in the pursuit of the PHG of relatedness. As it develops, the intervention plan can be reviewed against findings from a protective factor assessment in order to cross-check whether the plan considers relevant strengths that need to be sustained and developed. In this way, the rehabilitation plan is grounded in an individualized case formulation and checked against empirically identified composite constructs associated (but not necessarily causally) with desistance from crime.

3.5 Case Illustration: A GLM-Grounded Assessment

Here we illustrate application of a GLM-grounded assessment with a composite case example "Kane." Kane was a 37-year-old New Zealand Māori (indigenous) man imprisoned for the abduction and rape of a 15-year-old girl who was unknown to him, when he was 26 years old. Kane was sentenced to preventive detention (an indeterminate sentence) with a minimum non-parole period of 12 years. At the time of assessment, Kane was 10.5 years into his prison sentence and soon to begin a high-intensity sexual offense-focused treatment program. His Static-99R score placed him in the well above average risk category for sexual reoffending, hence his referral to a high-intensity program. The assessment was intended to identify relevant therapy needs. The following sections begin with an overview of relevant background information contained within official documentation and prison records. Next is a summary of key GLM-related assessment considerations, including identification of PHGs implicated in offending and those prioritized by Kane, and an exploration of obstacles to goods attainment. We then present a tentative GLM-grounded case formulation and intervention plan.

3.5.1 Background Information

Kane was removed from his mother when he was 5 years old by the state, and had never met his father. He transitioned through various foster homes and was physically and sexually abused by carers on multiple occasions. Kane ran away from foster care and joined a gang when he was 15 years old, becoming a well-respected senior gang member. Official records documented an extensive history of prior offending: 40 convictions for general and violent offending, including threatening to kill, male assaults on female, common assault, aggravated robbery, theft, and numerous driving-related offenses. Kane held no formal qualifications and had never held a legitimate job. He was on parole for aggravated robbery at the time of his index offending, prior to which he was reportedly attempting a fresh start away from gang associates with support from a local church.

Kane received several sanctions for misconduct early in his prison sentence, including escaping custody; however, he had not received any conduct reports in the 2 years preceding his assessment. Kane was transferred to his current unit 4 months ago. Soon after his arrival, Kane met and developed a positive rapport with a cultural support worker. The cultural support worker introduced Kane to traditional wood carving, and Kane was spending much of his free time carving and painting. In the sections that follow, we present GLM-specific assessment considerations, namely, the identification of PHGs (implicated in offending and prioritized currently), an exploration of obstacles experienced seeking out PHGs (supplemented by an assessment of protective factors), and good life goals.

3.5.2 Assessment of Primary Human Goods

Assessment commenced with an exploration of Kane's current concerns and life priorities. He spoke at length about his recently developed interests in *Te Ao Māori* (the Māori world) since engaging with the cultural support worker assigned to his unit. Kane reported that although he was Māori he'd never engaged with his culture, and until recently, he'd seen nothing good about being Māori. Now, for the first time in his life, he was learning about his cultural heritage and integrating being Māori into his self-concept. Kane had joined the unit's *kapahaka* (Māori performing arts) group through which he was developing friendships with peers from similar backgrounds to his own, and he was enjoying the unit's weekly volleyball tournaments. Kane excelled at sports and his talents were quickly recognized by his peers, making him a sought-after team member. When asked his sexual interests, Kane acknowledged lacking any template for consenting sex and openly discussed that the women in his life had served just one purpose: his own sexual gratification. He acknowledged ongoing masturbation to violent sexual fantasies, which he said provided him with a sense of empowerment. Kane's prioritized PHGs and his current means for seeking these are summarized in Table 3.1, listed in the general order they were identified. At the time of assessment, Kane demonstrated several adaptive secondary goods (means), along with several maladaptive secondary goods that put him at risk of ongoing offending in the absence of prosocial, adaptive, and personally meaningful alternatives.

Kane's report of his index offending was generally consistent with file information. When asked how he made sense of his offending, he reported it "just happened." He shared that in the months preceding his offending he had developed a connection with a similar-aged woman through the church he was receiving support from while on parole. He acknowledged she was the only reason he was attempting to distance himself from the gang and involve himself in church life. Kane described automatic

Table 3.1 Kane's prioritized primary human goods and pretreatment means

Primary good	Current means (secondary goods)
Creativity	Singing and playing guitar, wood carving, painting
Mastery in Play	Volleyball, wood carving
Community	Engagement with cultural support worker, member of *kapahaka*[a] group, senior gang member
Relatedness	Developing friendships through *kapahaka*[a] group, long-term friendships with fellow gang members
Agency	Verbal aggression, masturbation to rape fantasies
States of Happiness and Pleasure	Volleyball, gym sessions, masturbation to rape fantasies

[a]Māori performing arts

thoughts of "WTF" upon learning that she was not interested in progressing their relationship beyond a friendship. He promptly moved out of the accommodation the church was providing and returned immediately to his previous way of life and what he knew. He stated that soon after returning to a gang residence, he was driving around town and wanting sex. As soon as he found a woman walking alone who he found physically attractive, he abducted her, drove to a remote location, and raped her. Kane described feeling empowered and back in control of his life following his offending. Several PHGs were implicated in Kane's offending, notably agency and states of happiness and pleasure (which includes sexual pleasure).

3.5.3 Exploration of Obstacles to Goods Attainment

Kane demonstrated some insight into problems with both internal and external capacity he experienced throughout his life that had resulted in him joining a gang at 15 years old, and more recently, the challenges he faced in distancing himself from the gang and attempting a different life. Asked about what had gotten in the way of previous attempts to change, he reflected that he had nothing in common with the church volunteers. He stated that his developing friendship with the woman he met through the church was his only glimmer of hope, and one that was quickly quashed. Kane described feeling rejected by the woman, which triggered longstanding feelings of rejection from his mother. When asked how he coped with negative emotional states, Kane reported he had a short fuse and went into autopilot—often turning to aggression, substance use, and violent sex. SAPROF-SO ratings offered further insight into problems with capacity. Table 3.2 provides Kane's pretreatment SAPROF-SO ratings and brief scoring rationales. Each item is rated on a five-point scale, with zero indicating absent–low protection, one indicating low–moderate protection, two indicating moderate protection, three indicating moderate–high protection, and four indicating high protection.

Kane demonstrated an absent-to-low level of protection from the Resilience and Adaptive Sexuality items, and low-to-moderate protection from the Prosocial

Table 3.2 Kane's pretreatment protective factors ratings

SAPROF-SO scale/item	Scoring rationale	Score
Resilience		
1. Adaptive schemas	Longstanding borderline traits and beliefs other people can't be trusted (although recent engagement with cultural support worker had positive impact). Presents as self-confident, acknowledges mood fluctuates. Adaptive schemas dominant for past 3–4 months. Within past 12 months, maladaptive schemas activated frequently	1
2. Empathy	Encouraged a peer who risked being removed from the therapy unit for aggressive behavior to consider engaging with cultural support, sharing how helpful he was finding it. Empathy evident in one setting. No evidence of major failures to demonstrate empathy in past 6 months	1
3. Coping	Wood carving has become a positive outlet for anger. Struggles when carving is not accessible, acknowledges he has a short fuse, and is easily triggered. Examples of externalizing behavior (verbal aggression) evident in past 6 months	1
4. Self-control	Longstanding history of getting into fights, described self as mellowed in recent years; however, acknowledges occasional verbal altercations in past 12 months. No incident reports. Able to restrain self from getting into a fight	2
5. Attitudes toward rules and regulations	Compliant with prison rules; negative attitudes toward specific prison officers he perceives as racist and power hungry, expresses some resentment	2
	Resilience Average	1.4
	Adaptive Sexuality	
6. Sexual self-regulation	Normative sex drive (masturbates 2–3 times/week). Acknowledges fantasizing to rape themes which were reinforced in the gang. Acknowledges lacking a template for consenting adult sex. No evidence for any of the four elements of sexual self-regulation	0
7. Prosocial sexual interests	Dominant fantasies involve forced sex and feeling in control	0
8. Prosocial sexual identity	Reports heterosexual orientation, all previous sexual partners female (mostly adult, acknowledges some were underage, but "fully developed"). Given 0 on previous item, 0 indicated here (does not demonstrate prosocial sexual interests therefore cannot demonstrate prosocial sexual identity)	0
9. Intimate relationship	Not present	0
	Adaptive Sexuality Average	0
	Prosocial Connection and Reward	
10. Goal-directed living	Keen to learn more about his culture, engaged with cultural supports, enjoying wood carving and *kapahaka* (Māori performing arts) in spare time. Goals motivate prosocial behavior in stable and consistent way, they counteract major risk factors (antisocial peers) and provide a source of several primary goods (knowledge, community, relatedness). Goal-directed behavior relatively recent but consistent for past 4 months (approx.)	3

(continued)

Table 3.2 (continued)

SAPROF-SO scale/item	Scoring rationale	Score
11. Work	Works in prison workshop 16 h/week (max number of hours available to him). Valued by workshop manager. Acknowledges job is a good fit for him, although he'd prefer to have more autonomy and be more creative (vs. fulfill orders). Not resentful. States would rather be working than not as it helps kill time	2
12. Leisure activities	Kapakapa group—meets weekly. Regularly scheduled, enjoyable, likely with a mix of prosocial and antisocial peers given he's in prison	2
13. Social network	Since engagement in *kapahaka* has formed friendships with prosocial peers, including treatment program graduates. Net effect minimal given these friendships are relatively new. Kane has not shared much about himself with them but is beginning to trust them	1
14. Emotional connection to adults	Longstanding distrust of people outside his gang. No emotional connections identified at time of assessment	0
	Prosocial Connection and Reward Average	1.6
	Average SAPROF-SO score	1.07

Note. SAPROF-SO = Structured Assessment of PROtective Factors against Sexual Offending (Willis et al., 2022). SAPROF-SO items are rated 0–4 with higher scores associated with higher levels of protection

Connection and Reward items. The Resilience and Adaptive Sexuality items infer problems with internal capacity, including maladaptive schemas and coping skills. His stronger protection on the Prosocial Connection and Reward subscale was attributed largely to his recent engagement in *Te Ao Māori*, made possible through opportunities available to him in his current environment (e.g., cultural support worker, *kapahaka* group).

3.5.4 Tentative Case Formulation

The final stage of assessment involves integrating assessment data into a tentative case formulation which is updated as new information is shared. What follows is a working formulation based on data collected about Kane.

Kane was a 37-year-old man of Māori descent in prison for the abduction and rape of a 15-year-old girl who was unknown to him. An early learning environment grounded in cultural and intergenerational trauma left Kane distrustful of others and needing to fight for survival, including to escape abusive foster care environments. He found connection and a sense of belonging with men of similar backgrounds in a gang. The gang became a core part of his identity and a source for many PHGs, including relatedness, community, mastery (in work and play), states of happiness and pleasure, and agency. Violence toward women was normalized, and Kane lacked any template for consenting adult sex.

Following his last prison sentence, Kane contemplated a life outside the gang and was supported by a local church while on parole. Precipitating his index offending, however, perceived rejection from a potential romantic partner reignited several maladaptive schemas, including entrenched hostile beliefs about women. Kane felt despondent about his attempt for a different life. In the absence of adaptive means for coping with emotional distress (PHG: inner peace), Kane withdrew from prosocial supports and increasingly associated with the gang. On the day of his index offending, he was driving around town and wanting sex. As soon as he saw a woman he found attractive he coerced her into his car and drove to a remote location where he sexually assaulted her. Kane's offending gave him a sense of control (PHG: agency) and pleasure (PHG: states of happiness and pleasure) in an otherwise unpredictable world.

Kane is again contemplating life outside the gang. His recent engagement with cultural supports and activities represent key protective factors, providing sources of several PHGs previously acquired through the gang, including relatedness, community, and mastery in play.

3.5.5 Intervention/Therapy Planning

Kane's intervention plan provides the foundations for a future-oriented GLP and roadmap for the dual aims of GLM-grounded rehabilitation: Risk reduction and well-being enhancement. Intervention planning centers around Kane's good life goals as they relate to PHGs prioritized currently, and those implicated in his offending. The following clinician–client dialogue illustrates the process of identifying some of Kane's good life goals and those strengths in need of developing to realize them:

Therapist: "When you think of your life five years from now, what would be the ideal?"

Kane: "Ideal? Well, the ideal feels impossible outside these walls, but I dream about keeping on doing what I'm doing now, carving and painting, maybe someday making a living creating art for others."

Therapist: "And if you were making a living from your art, then what would you have?"

Kane: "I'd be spending my time doing something good. Doing something that makes me feel good, gives me focus, and when I'm creating my own work—a sense of freedom. Maybe it will help me connect with other Māori like me. And if I can get job out of it ... well maybe then I could afford to rent my own place one day."

Therapist: "Your carving and painting have many layers of meaning, they bring you joy, independence, and a sense of connection to your culture; and clearly you're very good at what you do. Your carving and painting seem to give you a sense of meaning and purpose...as the gang once did?"

Kane: "Yeah, they do, but life on the outside is so different to life here. Shit happens that you can't control, and it's so easy going back to what you know best."

Therapist: "That makes full sense. From what you've shared, it would seem your life has been unpredictable. Things have happened outside your control, and you've coped the best way you could, based on what you know. At the same time, it would seem that you have more motivation now than in the past for a different life. Would that be fair?"

Kane: "Yeah, there's definitely more motivation, more reason to leave the gang and these revolving doors."

Therapist: "This program will help support you to develop the strengths you need to deal with unknowns, and stay focused on the better life you want for yourself. When you think of that better life, painting and carving, feeling a sense of connection to your culture, having your independence....what obstacles do you see getting in the way on the outside?"

Kane: "There are many. The gang has been my life—my family, my friends, the roof over my head. Without anyone else, well it would be bloody hard not to go back. I don't know any different. I don't know how to get a job. I don't know how to date a woman. And I sure as hell don't know how to be intimate with a woman."

Therapist: "The gang has been a way of life, and contemplating anything different is scary. You've learned ways of living in the gang. And you can learn different ways of living. We don't want to set you up for failure, we want to help you develop skills that will help keep you on track towards that better life. You've identified some areas we can focus on in therapy, including coping with unknowns, and strengthening your knowledge and skills surrounding intimate relationships."

As illustrated in the therapist–client dialogue, Kane's initial good life goals included having friends outside gangs, relating better to women, and continuing with his carving and painting. Kane's good life goals identified following assessment are listed in Table 3.3, alongside associated strengths in need of development to achieve these goals.

The four good life goals listed in Table 3.3 provide sources of multiple PHGs: Having friends outside gangs aligns with the primary goods of relatedness and community; relating better to women aligns with the primary goods of relatedness and states of happiness and pleasure; continuing carving and painting aligns with agency, mastery in play, mastery in work, and creativity; and finding calmness relates to inner peace. A review of Table 3.3 against SAPROF-SO ratings in Table 3.2 suggests key strengths in need of development were accounted for. In particular, there was a focus on developing sexual self-regulation skills and prosocial sexual interests, strengthening adaptive schemas, and strengthening connections to prosocial peers and networks. Kane's SAPROF-SO ratings provide a baseline from which therapy progress can be assessed. As Kane's capacity for working toward good life goals strengthens, so too will his protective factor ratings. Thus, rerating a measure

Table 3.3 Kane's good life goals and strengths in need of development

Good life goals	Strengths to develop (therapy goals)
Have friends outside gangs	• Strengthen connections with prosocial peers • Strengthen connections with cultural supports
Relate better to women, have a healthy relationship one day	• Address distrust and hostility toward women • Develop fantasies for consenting adult sex • Reinforcement of consenting fantasies
Continue carving and painting on release	• Develop connections with cultural supports in the community • Develop coping skills for dealing with unknowns
Find calmness in my life	• Develop adaptive ways of managing emotions without reliance on sex

of protective factors can provide an indication for the extent to which clients have developed capacities to implement a prosocial GLP.

3.6 Conclusion

This chapter has described and illustrated key considerations for implementing the GLM in pretreatment clinical assessments alongside RNR considerations. Implementing the GLM from initial client contact and throughout the assessment process capitalizes on opportunities to engage clients at the earliest opportunity, helping them recognize that ultimately treatment goals align with their own life goals. Clients in treatment "…want better lives not simply the promise of less harmful ones" (Ward et al., 2007, p. 106). An early focus on risk reduction alone carries the risk of clients being passive recipients of interventions that follow, and is a poor use of correctional resources. Instead, identifying a person's prioritized PHGs and their expression in their practical identity and daily life provides important information for engaging clients in the process of change. Only when clients are engaged will correctional rehabilitation achieve its primary aim of preventing future victimization.

References

Barnao, M. (2013). The Good Lives Model tool kit for mentally disordered offenders. *The Journal of Forensic Practice, 15*, 157–170. https://doi.org/10.1108/JFP-07-2012-0001

Bonta, J., & Andrews, D. A. (2017). *The psychology of criminal conduct* (6th ed.). Routledge.

de Vogel, V., de Ruiter, C., Bouman, Y., & de Vries Robbé, M. (2012). *SAPROF. Guidelines for the assessment of protective factors for violence risk* (2nd ed.). Van der Hoeven Stichting.

Fernandez, Y. M., Harris, A. J. R., Hanson, R. K., & Sparks, J. (2014). *Stable-2007 Coding Manual – Revised 2014*. Unpublished report. Public Safety Canada.

Gannon, T. A., & Ward, T. (2014). Where has all the psychology gone? A critical review of evidence-based psychological practice in correctional settings. *Aggression and Violent Behavior, 19*, 435–446. https://doi.org/10.1016/j.avb.2014.06.006

Hanson, R. K., Harris, A. J. R., Scott, T., & Helmus, L. (2007). *Assessing the risk of sexual offenders on community supervision: The Dynamic Supervision Project* (Corrections Research User Report No. 2007-05). Public Safety Canada.

Heffernan, R., Ward, T., Vandevelde, S., & Van Damme, L. (2019). Dynamic risk factors and constructing explanations of offending: The Risk-Causality method. *Aggression and Violent Behavior, 44*, 47–56. https://doi.org/10.1016/j.avb.2018.11.009

Levenson, J. S., & Willis, G. M. (2019). Implementing trauma-informed care in correctional treatment and supervision. *Journal of Aggression, Maltreatment & Trauma, 28*(4), 481–501. https://doi.org/10.1080/10926771.2018.1531959

Levenson, J. S., Willis, G. M., & Prescott, D. S. (2017). *Trauma-informed care: Transforming treatment for people who have sexually abused*. Safer Society Press.

Prescott, D. S., & Willis, G. M. (2021). Using the Good Lives Model (GLM) in clinical practice: Lessons learned from international implementation projects. *Aggression and Violent Behavior, 63*, 101717. https://doi.org/10.1016/j.avb.2021.101717

Print, B. (Ed.). (2013). *The Good Lives Model for adolescents who sexually harm*. Safer Society Press.
Purvis, M., Ward, T., & Shaw, S. (2013). *Applying the Good Lives Model to the case management of sexual offenders*. Safer Society Press.
Purvis, M., Ward, T., & Willis, G. M. (2011). The Good Lives Model in practice: Offence pathways and case management. *European Journal of Probation, 3*(2), 4–28.
Taylor, E. (2017). 'I should have been a security consultant': The Good Lives Model and residential burglars. *European Journal of Criminology, 14*, 434–450. https://doi.org/10.1177/1477370816661743
Vess, J., Ward, T., & Collie, R. (2008). Case formulation with sex offenders: An illustration of individualized risk assessment. *The Journal of Behavior Analysis of Offender and Victim Treatment and Prevention, 1*(3), 284–293. https://doi.org/10.1037/h0100450
Wanzeele, W., & Seys, A. (2023). Mensen die seksueel grensoverschrijdend gedrag ontkennen: Aan de slag met het Good Lives Model. *Tijdschrift voor Forensische Psychiatrie en Psychologie, 1*(1), 89–104. https://doi.org/10.5553/TFPP/295044302023001001006
Ward, T. (2016). Dynamic risk factors: Scientific kinds or predictive constructs. *Psychology, Crime & Law, 22*, 2–16. https://doi.org/10.1080/1068316X.2015.1109094
Ward, T. (2017). Prediction and agency: The role of protective factors in correctional rehabilitation and desistance. *Aggression and Violent Behavior, 32*, 19–28. https://doi.org/10.1016/j.avb.2016.11.012
Ward, T., Clack, S., & Haig, B. D. (2017). The abductive theory of method: Scientific inquiry and clinical practice. *Behaviour Change, 33*, 212–231. https://doi.org/10.1017/bec.2017.1
Ward, T., Mann, R. E., & Gannon, T. A. (2007). The good lives model of offender rehabilitation: Clinical implications. *Aggression and Violent Behavior, 12*, 87–107. https://doi.org/10.1016/j.avb.2006.03.004
Willis, G. M., Kelley, S. M., Thornton, D., Tucker, M., & Smolinski, T. (2024). *Can the SAPROF-SO replace dynamic risk tools to help inform therapy goals?* Manuscript submitted for publication.
Willis, G. M., Thornton, D., Kelley, S. M., & de Vries Robbé, M. (2022). *The Structured Assessment of Protective Factors against Sexual Offending (SAPROF-SO) V1 Manual*. Figshare. https://doi.org/10.17608/k6.auckland.19251899.v1
Willis, G. M., Ward, T., & Levenson, J. S. (2014). The Good Lives Model (GLM): An evaluation of GLM operationalization in North American treatment programs. *Sexual Abuse, 26*, 58–81. https://doi.org/10.1177/1079063213478202
Wong, S., Olver, M. E., Nicholaichuk, T. P., & Gordon, A. (2003–2017). *The Violence Risk Scale: Sexual Offense version (VRS-SO)*. Regional Psychiatric Centre and University of Saskatchewan.
Yates, P. M., Kingston, D. A., & Ward, T. (2009). *The Self-Regulation Model of the offence and re-offence process: A guide to assessment and treatment planning using the integrated Good Lives/Self-Regulation Model of sexual offending*. Pacific Psychological Assessment Corporation.
Yates, P. M., Prescott, D. S., & Ward, T. (2010). *Applying the Good Lives and Self Regulation Models to sex offender treatment: A practical guide for clinicians*. Safer Society Press.

Chapter 4
Intervention Framework and Issues

4.1 Introduction

This chapter examines how to (and how not to) apply GLM treatment interventions. In line with the description of evidence-based practices in Chap. 1, it builds on clinical experience from implementation projects around the world, reviews research-based best practice in program implementation, and offers guidance on matching treatment services to client characteristics, preferences, and cultural considerations (effective GLM intervention requires that the latter be considered in both assessment and treatment). While Chap. 1 includes a more comprehensive overview of the theoretical underpinnings and discussion of the three levels of the GLM, this chapter explores their application in practice settings.

In brief, GLM interventions center on a personally meaningful good life plan, containing all primary goods to varying degrees (chosen by the individual), and the secondary goods (goals and strategies) required to attain these without harming others (Ward et al., 2024). This can be linked with risk reduction by identification of the goods sought via offending (either directly or indirectly) in the past, and the barriers or problems (i.e., criminogenic needs as motivational signals) evident within the strategies used to attain these goods. For example, sexual offending is sometimes used to achieve relatedness or pleasure because of problems differentiating between appropriate partners (i.e., children are preferred as sexual partners because individuals feel emotionally safer with them). A treatment good life plan could incorporate relatedness and pleasure via the goal of seeking an intimate relationship with an age-appropriate consenting partner. Treatment strategies may include attending social activities, creating an online dating profile, engaging in conversation, physical intimacy, vulnerable disclosure, conflict resolution, and so on. Treatment can target risk factors, such as emotional congruence with children, through the development or strengthening of internal and external capacities and resources. For example, developing healthy beliefs about the self, others, and relationships (e.g.,

T. Ward et al., *The Good Lives Model of Correctional Rehabilitation*,
Advances in Preventing and Treating Violence and Aggression,
https://doi.org/10.1007/978-3-031-95559-4_4

"others are trustworthy," "I am safe"), communication and negotiation skills, emotion management, perspective-taking, and so on. The availability of external resources (e.g., opportunity, finances, freedom) can support or obstruct PHG attainment and should also be included in a good life plan.

Essentially, GLM-guided treatment should identify the most heavily weighted goods (which are linked to a person's practical identity and sense of meaning) and those sought via offending, use these to construct a comprehensive good life plan, and then develop or strengthen the internal and external resources required to live a good life without reoffending. The GLM proposes a dual focus on promoting goods and overcoming internal and external barriers. It does this in collaboration with the individual to build on strengths and focus on meaningful personal goals, rather than simply avoiding reoffending.

The GLM has been used in a wide variety of ways in diverse settings on virtually every continent with very different populations. These settings include prisons, psychiatric hospitals, special commitment centers, intensive residential programs, group homes, and community-based treatment programs. While this provides testimony to the adaptability of the GLM, it also means that there are misunderstandings about what the GLM actually is and how it should be applied (Ward et al., 2024).

4.2 What the GLM Is and What It Is Not

Since its introduction, many programs and practitioners have implemented the GLM in diverse ways, sometimes more successfully than others. Chapter 1 describes three interwoven levels of the GLM: core values, knowledge-related assumptions, and practice guidelines. It is worthwhile for practitioners to bear in mind these levels when considering individual clients or implementation of the GLM in a program or constellation of programs. Using the three levels as a backdrop, it is critical that before applying the GLM, programs and practitioners should:

- Be grounded in mission of building internal and external capacities for clients.
- Pay equal attention to risk variables.
- Keep in mind that the overall focus of the GLM is to help clients achieve well-being and a life worth living as well as in managing risk.
- Consider that client successes often stem from the interactive nature of this dual emphasis. Clients who are seeking to live a better life often find managing risk easier to accomplish than if their sole focus is on avoiding reoffending.
- Approach each client as a fellow human being in the world rather than little more than the sum of their risk factors. Each client has fundamental human rights and is worthy of dignity and respect.
- Strive to remain strengths-based in every area of intervention. Programs and practitioners that do not have a strengths-based perspective will not be successful with the GLM.
- Understand that human beings are goal-directed and autonomous, and their behavior is meaningful and with purpose.

The points above are worth emphasizing because programs can often lose sight of them. Programs have sometimes relegated pieces of the GLM to psychoeducational module, as if saying, "Here is a list of goals (referring to the primary human goods [PHGs]) you might accomplish once you are done taking responsibility for your actions and are managing your risk factors." Having a firm foundation in the three interwoven levels can prevent misapplication of the model further.

As programs seek to implement the GLM, it can be useful to begin by reviewing their goals. Programs commonly have a mission statement that is explicitly written in policy and often reflected in the culture of the program. For example, many programs in the USA have a mission statement along the lines of, "no more victims." While this is a laudable goal on its face and no professional in this work wishes for people to be victimized, it does not align with the foundation of the GLM. In some cases, programs with a no-more-victims mission have explicitly or inadvertently veered away from the evidence for what works in preventing further offending. These programs have focused so much on risk management that they have forgotten the other side of the equation: that people who work to lead better lives are more likely to be successful in leading fulfilled, offense-free lives. In part, this is because individuals who commit offenses are motivated by a set of fundamental human desires (PHG) and therefore seek to achieve goals such as intimacy, a sense of control, or social acceptance rather than simply an offense. In these cases, a mission along the lines of, "preventing further victimization by ensuring that clients build lives that are incompatible with offending" might be more useful.

Over time, several misconceptions about the GLM have become apparent during GLM training and consultation efforts, which are useful to address early on:

- The GLM is a practice framework and not a specific treatment protocol (see Chap. 1). Many programs and practitioners have come to assume that the GLM must be like the empirically supported protocols (ESTs) that they have learned in other settings and that are emphasized in contemporary public discourse. Dialectical behavior therapy (Linehan, 2014), for example, requires very strict adherence to a set of methods. Those using motivational interviewing are often trained to use certain behavior counts, such as maintaining a ratio of two reflective statements for every open-ended question asked. Other ESTs are modularized in a specific sequence. These approaches often have an excellent research base and are worthy of the term EST. There are good reasons to employ each of these methods and models; indeed, many of their techniques blend well with the GLM. However, the emphasis on ESTs in various locations around the world has often meant that the flexibility of the GLM practice framework requires a fresh perspective on how treatment works.
- Keeping the above in mind, the GLM is not time limited. Program administrators interested in learning about the model frequently ask how long or how many sessions it takes. The duration of treatment will depend on the individual and the nature of ancillary treatment needs (for example, see the case example of Linda in Chap. 8. In her case, treating her substance abuse disorder would be a major component of her treatment.) While programs will wish to be familiar with available literature on treatment dosage, the course of GLM treatment should be determined by the individual's risks and needs).

- The GLM is not designed to be implemented in any one specific or inflexible way. However, some elements are essential in any successful implementation, and these are described below.
- Further, there is no official certification of GLM practitioners or programs. There are many reasons for this, including the absence of a research base showing that certification efforts improve outcomes for clients. Rather, the authors recommend that programs and practitioners adhere to the findings of implementation studies (e.g., Fixsen et al., 2005). This includes reading the extant literature, attending training, receiving consultation, using the fidelity monitoring tool mentioned later in this chapter, and establishing deliberate practice plans (Prescott et al., 2017) to ensure that their skills are improving.
- Properly applied, the GLM is not a way of telling clients what is wrong or missing from their lives. Some practitioners have taken a reductionistic view of the GLM and have expressed the view that, at its core, the GLM is simply a way of reminding clients what's wrong with them. This view reflects a deep misunderstanding of the GLM as an overarching practice framework. Therapists should not view themselves as normative police officers, always searching for value violations and correcting clients. Practitioners reminding clients of what is wrong or missing from their lives are not practicing the GLM.
- Properly applied, the GLM is not patronizing or paternalistic. While some have rightly warned against this in the literature (Glaser, 2011), its focus is on viewing the client as a fellow traveler and relies heavily on the therapist characteristics described below. Care must be taken to elicit honest feedback from the client on what is and isn't working in therapy, and what they need more or less of. Goals related to well-being should never be imposed on a client but should result from clinical discussion.
- The GLM is not "done to" a client. The GLM is inherently collaborative.

In summary, the GLM applied properly is delivered in a collaborative manner, builds on client strengths, and depends on understanding and responding to clients' personal and cultural values alongside their histories of adverse experiences.

4.3 A Note on Coercive Approaches and Treatment Experience

It is worth noting that research has consistently found that the greater the level of coercion experienced in treatment, the less likely these services are to be effective at reducing recidivism (Parhar et al., 2008). In some corners of the world, intrusive and invasive methods such as aversion therapy using noxious smells, the penile plethysmograph, and polygraph examinations have often played a role in assessment and treatment. Each of these has been controversial in the literature for many reasons, and a full accounting is well beyond the scope of this book.

Historically, writings on the GLM have been silent regarding these methods. While some jurisdictions have required the use of the polygraph as a condition of probation, but when used against the client's wishes, these methods are antithetical to the core values of the GLM. It may be useful to clarify this with clients in the service of the therapeutic relationship. Nevertheless, many practitioners using the GLM have found themselves with no choice (for example, a probation department requires a polygraph examination if the client wants to live freely in the community as opposed to in an institution). Under these circumstances, practitioners should regard these methods as outside the core values and scope of the GLM practice framework, and special care may be needed to reduce any harm that may result.

4.4 Therapist Characteristics

Attention to therapist characteristics is essential in the GLM framework; this section offers ideas to help operationalize them. Empirical attention to therapist characteristics and treatment process variables has emerged since the 1990s (Drapeau, 2005; Marshall, 2005; Miller & Rollnick, 2023). To summarize, Marshall (2005) reviewed the available research, including in forensic treatment programs, and outlined that the most effective therapists were those who are:

- Warm
- Empathic
- Rewarding
- Directive

"Directive" in this case means having a clear sense of direction and moving treatment forward accordingly. Together, these characteristics form the acronym WERD, which helps people newer to the field to remember them. It is important to recognize that no one is always at their best at displaying these features in every personal and professional setting, and so each of these can be the focus of ongoing "deliberate practice" efforts (Chow, 2017).

Along similar lines, a large body of motivational interviewing research (Miller & Rollnick, 2023) has illustrated the importance of the "spirit" of motivational interviewing (sometimes also thought of as its mindset and heart set). This involves interacting with each client in a spirit of:

- Partnership
- Acceptance
- Compassion
- Empowerment

To accomplish this, Miller and Rollnick (2023) emphasize the importance of approaching each client with humility; the practitioner may be an expert in the forensic arena, but only the client is the ultimate expert on their life. These central values form the acronym PACE, which can also be a useful acronym to help newer practitioners stay grounded.

Attention to each of these variables and the core values, knowledge assumptions, and practice guidelines form the foundation of the GLM. Sadly, research has found that therapists can overestimate their effectiveness with clients (Beech & Fordham, 1997; Levenson et al., 2024; Walfish et al., 2012). For this reason, it is vital that practitioners get ongoing feedback from their clients on what is and isn't working for them (Prescott et al., 2022a, 2022b). Together, the above characteristics provide a firm foundation for therapists working with the GLM.

4.5 Approach Versus Avoidance Goals

Approach and avoidance goals are introduced in Chap. 1. These types of goals have to do with whether a person is approaching a goal that they can achieve, attain, or acquire, or that they otherwise aspire to as opposed to something they are simply trying to avoid. Examples of approach goals from daily life include developing healthier eating habits, improving relationships, or spending more time feeling at peace. Examples of avoidance goals might be to not eat unhealthy foods, stay away from friends who aren't good for them, and feeling less stressed out. The way that people frame their goals can help determine whether they are successful. Approaching better physical health can be a more appealing goal than quitting smoking.

The practitioner's work involves managing the delicate balance between the approach goal of promoting the individual's goods and the avoidance goal of reducing risk. For the purposes of treatment planning and practices, it is important to bear in mind that the PHGs and development of a good life plan rely in large part on the use of approach goals. This can be a difficult challenge for newer practitioners who are often used to thinking in terms of reducing symptoms, solving problems, fixing that which is broken, or making others stop their harmful behaviors.

Professionals occasionally raise the concern that approach goals might not be a good fit with a particular client. For example, they may ask whether the client who says, "My only goal at present is to avoid further offending" shouldn't be allowed to retain this as a goal. This question typically arises as a hypothetical, and the authors have never heard of a case in which avoiding offending was in fact the only aspiration that the client had. In these cases, the therapist or evaluator might:

- Simply have a conversation with the client to see what other aspirations arise and how they might connect to their good life plan at the time of their offending or in their future. This could involve asking clients why they want to avoid offending, what's stopping them from having and doing what they want in their lives, and what they would gain if they did put an end to harmful behaviors. This might help to elucidate other goals.
- Begin treatment with the central goal being to avoid offending and using sessions to understand what the client's good life plan was at the time of their harmful behavior. As therapy proceeds, the client may come to view their life as a mix of approach and avoidance goals, then work to reorganize their plans accordingly. Remember, offending provides a window into clients prioritized PHGs and associated practical identities (see Chaps. 1 and 2).

What programs and practitioners should never do is tell them that an avoidance-based goal is not allowed or insist that the client must fit themselves into the GLM before they are ready. As a colleague once asked in a training about empirically supported protocols, "Are we personalizing our manuals or are we trying to manualize persons?" These are all reasons why the GLM is a practice framework and not a specific protocol.

4.6 Getting the Context Right

Some additional considerations for getting started with the GLM include:

- The therapist's grounding in the agent-action-context schema mentioned in Chap. 1. This can help therapists keep focused on the many components involved in problematic behaviors and not just the actions or characteristics of the agent.
- Taking client concerns seriously and listening for evidence of the PHGs behind the concern. For example, the client who doubts whether a program or practitioner can help them is likely expressing concerns about internal and external capacities involving the PHG of relatedness.
- Likewise, listening for evidence of early life adversity when clients are expressing concerns can help to foment an understanding.
- For clients residing in a secure setting or under intensive community monitoring for more than a year into the future, it may be helpful to consider developing intervention plans both for while the client is residing in the high-intensity setting and again as they are approaching a return to greater freedom in the community.
- In inpatient settings, it is helpful to have the paraprofessional and/or security staff trained to have familiarity with the model so that they can provide support to clients (also see Chap. 10). In some non-forensic inpatient settings, such as group homes (see the case of Linda in Chap. 8), there may be activities or psychoeducational groups that the paraprofessional staff can provide.
- Consider the language used. This book and virtually all the other GLM literature use the term "primary human goods," which many clients will find difficult to understand. Many GLM resources (e.g., Prescott & Pflugradt, 2024) use the term "good life goal" in its place (see Chap. 3). This kind of adaptation is not made lightly. It is vital to the integrity of the GLM that the PHGs be thought of by the practitioner as actions, experiences, and states of being that one seeks to attain for their own sake. This means that they are more than simply goals. However, when applying the model in forensic settings and other agencies, it can be helpful to operationalize the PHGs as goals. Likewise, it is worthwhile to remember that some words may have different connotations in various areas of the world. "Agency," for example, may need to be restated as "personal choice and independence" in some settings. Likewise, relatedness may be restated as "to love and be loved."[1]

---

[1] See Appendix F for suggestions for translating primary human goods into good life goals.

4.7 Getting Started

Once the formal assessment is complete (and the therapist and client understand the results, case conceptualization, and intervention plan), an excellent place to start when speaking with the client is to consider the components of the therapeutic alliance (Ross et al., 2008). While many therapists confuse this term with having a positive relationship with a client, the therapeutic alliance, as defined by Bordin (1979) and reconsidered more recently by Norcross (2010) is more comprehensive. As applied to the GLM, practitioners can ask:

- Do the client and I agree on the goals of therapy?
- Do the client and I agree on the nature of our relationship and how I fit into their life?
- Do the client and I agree on the approaches used in treatment?
- Are the client and I working in accordance with their cultural values and strongly held beliefs?

These questions, and the resulting feedback from clients, can yield insights into how and when clients may not move forward in treatment. As good as any assessment process may be, the final report may not fully convey the intricacies of a client's daily life, and therapists may not always see PHG-related content in sessions. For example:

Therapist (T): "Welcome, Chris! It's great to see you here today."
Client (C): "Well, it's not so great to see you today. They scheduled this session at the same time as I was supposed to work over in the machine shop, at the other end of this hellhole of a prison. No offense, but you're just about the last person I want to talk to right now."

For some therapists, this brief exchange might appear as resistance, and they may feel compelled to respond accordingly. After all, job opportunities can be plentiful, while therapy sessions need to be scheduled when they can. These therapists might be tempted to remind the client about the realities of treatment within a prison setting, such as scheduling challenges and the importance of treatment completion to establishing release dates. Some therapists might assume that the client is manipulating the therapist and trying to avoid treatment intervention. Still other therapists, seeking to be helpful, may start by attempting to resolve the scheduling conflict (which is an excellent idea, but may only offset a deeper and more compassionate response within the GLM framework).

Seen through the lens of the therapeutic alliance, several opportunities present themselves for a helpful intervention. Starting with the questions above:

Do the client and I agree on the goals of treatment? In this case, the client is providing a lesson about what is meaningful and important to them. First, the overall presentation reflects the client's concerns about agency. By all appearances, he wants to be in charge of how his life is balanced with respect to such elements as therapy and mastery experiences. He is angry at the impositions on his independence and autonomy in this situation. While the client's presentation may be rude, the compassionate therapist can see that this person is seeking out the very same agency that the staff of the prison take for granted. Further, in explicitly saying that the therapist is the last person that they want to see at that moment, the client is demonstrating that relatedness has a place in his life and that there is discord and possible rupture within the therapeutic relationship, whether either of them asked for it or not. Finally, the client is explicitly emphasizing the importance of mastery at work.

Do the client and I agree on the nature of our relationship? In the few words exchanged above are many possibilities for reflection. Does the client view the therapist as an agent of the police power of the state? As a tool of a cruel and unjust system? Are they simply another person in their life who wields undue influence over them? Or as someone who might help if only they really understood the client? Do they view the therapist as a source of shame or of support and validation? These may all be possible, and other more subtle differences may be present. Does the client think therapy is a place where they must express emotions all the time? Do they confuse the relationship they have with that of their mother, father, potential lover, etc? This will be very important to clarify, since the PHG of relatedness is so often central to clients' good life plans.

Do the client and I agree on the approaches used in treatment? In this instance, the client may be the therapist's best teacher. Through this brief exchange, the client is offering information as to what will and won't work. Treatment that honors the client's sense of agency and mastery at work will likely be the most successful. While the impulse to rush toward problem-solving is not misguided, it may overlook an opportunity for a broader discussion of how they can work together in the future.

Are the client and I working in accordance with their cultural values and strongly held beliefs? While there is no information about cultural values in the vignette above, the client is letting the therapist know about his strongly held values (mastery at work and agency). It seems that these PHGs are central to his *practical identity*, described in Chaps. 1 and 8. Proceeding with respect for this practical identity will serve the client and therapist well. It will help to prevent the client from developing a bleak outlook on his future and sense of meaning and purpose, which is connected to the PHG of spirituality. When programs introduce challenges to mastery at work for people to whom this is part of their practical identity, they have the rehabilitative process backward. When programs work to produce balance in change efforts and other activities, they are modeling the core values of the GLM.

Instead of responding with an immediate attempt to solve the problem or provide guidance on the role of the client, a better way forward would be:

T: "You're missing out on work right now and it's got you angry."

C: "Yes. It was in that assessment they did that work is important to me. Every hour matters. I need skills and I need to get out of here someday."

T: "We're about to figure out the best way forward. But first, can I just ask: Am I correct that it's not just about the hours and the pay and the skills. This is about who you are as a working man, and every roadblock is a potential threat to your autonomy and eventual independence, and even a bit about how you plan to live and survive?" (all PHGs).

C: (pausing and thinking):" Yes. Now let me ask you. What are you going to do about it?"

T: "The first thing I'm going to do is to get with your employer to work out our scheduling. Nothing's ever perfect when it comes to scheduling, but we will work something out. Anything I should know first, like are you a morning or a night person?"

C: "That part doesn't matter so much."

T: "Okay, I'll make a phone call in a moment, and you're invited to be part of it. First can I ask: We both know you're in prison and I'm a therapist. We both know this is my job and I go home at night. What I don't know is what you expect and what you hope for in working with me. What are your thoughts about how we work together? What else is important for me to know? What are your thoughts about how all this works?"

C: "That's a lot of questions."

T: 'How about this: How do you see me fitting into your life?"

C: "I don't know if I do see you fitting into my life."

T: "You're not sure you can trust any of this."

C: "No."

T: "So, you'll hear me out and take me at my word and then wait to see if I'm true to it all, correct?"

C: "Yes."

T: "Thanks. I'll keep working on it. Shall we call over to your work about that schedule?"

By listening reflectively, and with each of these components of the therapeutic alliance understood, the therapist has gained additional insights into how best to work with this client.

4.8 What Does the End of Treatment Look Like?

The GLM mapping tool and intervention plan referenced in Chap. 3 are excellent resources for assessment, understanding, and treatment. This section explores how they fit into the broader context of a treatment program. In real-world settings, it is often difficult for clients and practitioners alike to know what the expectations of treatment actually are, especially when programs are working within broader agencies of mental health or corrections and the legal systems beyond.

Understanding what is expected within the GLM framework is an important aspect of getting treatment started. Put another way, what does the end of treatment look like for the program and for the client? The answers often depend on the systems in which treatment occurs and are, therefore, all the more important to clarify. Clients who don't clearly understand the endpoint and what's expected of them often find themselves having difficulty moving forward in treatment programs and with their lives more generally.

Different settings will have different expectations and policies regarding expectations in treatment. Many inpatient settings require a comprehensive risk assessment to examine overall risk and potential next steps for a client. For clients residing in the community, treatment completion may be inextricably linked with decisions made by a case manager or probation officer. In some cases, a court hearing may be required so that a judge can lift a treatment requirement.

Some treatment programs follow a structure of three to four phases. The first phase focuses on addressing whatever aspects of the client's life might interfere with treatment. The second phase explores the client's past good life plan and helps them to develop internal and external capacities to begin working on a new good life plan. Subsequent work can explore how a client can build more horizontal and vertical coherence in their good life plan with a focus on their practical identity/identities. A third phase focuses on the implementation and refinement of the good life plan, while the fourth and final phase may represent a sort of aftercare situation, reviewing the ups and downs of the client's good life plan in daily life. In one instance, an inpatient program was clever and made clear in their policies that the aftercare phase, by definition, was to take place in the community. This ensured that the judges overseeing cases knew that leaving them in the institution was not an option. It also ensured that clients got the services they needed once they were out in the community.

In several sources (e.g., Prescott & Pflugradt, 2024), a series of questions can be useful for each PHG. These questions are intended for deep exploration and discussion for treatment planning, not simple answers:

4.9 Past

- What are all the ways that the client attempted to achieve this PHG in the past?
- What internal and external strengths and resources did they have to achieve this PHG?
- What worked and/or didn't work for them?
- How did the processes underlying risk play a role in this PHG?
- What challenges did they face?
- How did adverse and otherwise traumatic events act as roadblocks on the way to achieving this PHG?
- Looking back, did they overemphasize this PHG at the expense of others? Or did they neglect this PHG?
- What did they notice about their efforts when things were going well in attaining this PHG?
- What did others (close friends, family, or acquaintances) notice when things were going well for the client in attaining this PHG?

- Did they notice when things weren't working or were getting worse? If so, what did they notice?
- Did others notice when things weren't working? If so, what did they notice and how did they let the client know?
- Were there other sources of feedback, things that people said or did, that acted as warning signs when things were getting worse with respect to this PHG?
- How did they acknowledge progress or lack of progress in achieving this PHG? Did they ever celebrate this progress? If so, how?

4.10 Present

- What are all the ways that the client is currently attempting to achieve this PHG?
- What internal and external strengths and resources do they have to achieve this PHG?
- What's working and what's not working for them?
- How are the processes underlying risk playing a role in their current efforts to achieve this PHG?
- What challenges are they facing now?
- How are past adverse experiences and otherwise traumatic events continuing to act as roadblocks on the way to achieving this PHG?
- Are they overemphasizing this PHG at the expense of others? Or might they be neglecting it? How can they best ensure vertical and horizontal coherence?
- What do they notice about their efforts when things are going well in attaining this PHG?
- What do others notice when things are going well for this client in attaining this PHG?
- Does the client notice when things aren't working or are getting worse? If so, what do they notice?
- Do others in their life (close friends, family, or acquaintances) notice when things aren't working? If so, what do they notice and how did they let the client know?
- Are there other sources of feedback that act as warning signs that things are getting worse with respect to this PHG?
- How does the client acknowledge progress or lack of progress in achieving this PHG? Do they celebrate this progress? If so, how?

4.11 Future

- How does the client plan to achieve this PHG in the future?
- What internal and external strengths and resources will they have to achieve this PHG?

- What internal and external strengths and resources do they still need to develop to achieve this PHG?
- How might the processes underlying risk play a role in their future efforts to achieve this PHG?
- What challenges do they anticipate facing?
- How might the client's past adverse experiences and otherwise traumatic events act as roadblocks on the way to achieving this PHG and what would need to happen to prevent this?
- Are there ways that they might overemphasize this PHG at the expense of others? Or might they neglect it while focusing on other PHGs? What can they do to maintain vertical and horizontal coherence in their GLP going forward?
- What will they notice about their efforts when things are going well in attaining this PHG?
- What will others notice when things are going well for this client in attaining this PHG?
- What will the client notice when things aren't working or are getting worse? What ways will be available to them to take stock of what's working?
- What will others in their life (close friends, family, or acquaintances) notice when things aren't working? How can they let the client know?
- Are there other sources of feedback that will act as warning signs that things are getting worse with respect to this PHG?
- How will the client acknowledge progress or lack of progress in achieving this PHG? Do they celebrate this progress? If so, how?

Negotiating present and future good life plans can also involve discussions about how skills, circumstances, and vertical and horizontal coherence may change when someone is off intensive supervision in the community or leaves a high-security setting.

4.12 Understanding the Role of Trauma and Early Life Adversity

There has been a surge of research and practical interest in trauma-informed care in recent years (Levenson et al., 2017; Levenson & Willis, 2019). While a full description is beyond the scope of this chapter, a few points can be helpful for evaluators and therapists using the GLM.

First, it is important to distinguish trauma-specific treatment protocols (for example, eye movement desensitization and reprocessing; Shapiro, 2018) from trauma-informed care, which is best thought of as a set of principles that include understanding the impact that traumatic events have had on people's lives. Chapter 8 includes two cases of clients who have each been affected by trauma and adversity. The case example of Linda shows how a specific empirically supported protocol was used to address a long history of trauma and adversity. On the other hand, the case of Tommy includes discussion of how adversity was related to his practical identity and the PHGs implicated in his offense. Together, the cases illustrate how the effects of trauma can vary dramatically from one client to the next and that, just as in every aspect of the GLM, one size never fits all.

Second, the impact of complex trauma and its aftereffects can influence internal and external capacity for achieving PHGs. The effects of trauma and adversity often fall into three overarching domains: attachments and relationships, cognitions and core beliefs about the world, and self-regulation (Levenson et al., 2017). Looking at each, one can imagine many ways how each of these domains are affected:

Attachments and relationships. Problems in this area can prevent internal (and potentially external) capacity development in:

- Relatedness
- Community
- Living and surviving (through viewing relationships as a potential existential threat)
- Knowledge (via difficulties working with and trusting teachers and similar professionals)
- Mastery at play (through not being able to engage in activities with others)
- Mastery at work (by not being able to form collaborative relationships with colleagues)

Cognitions and core beliefs about the world. When the world is viewed as a dangerous or out-of-control place, where might makes right and authorities can't be trusted, it is no surprise that these kinds of cognitions could interfere with reaching one's full potential with respect to all of the PHGs. Related conditions might include two challenges to executive functioning often seen in people with long histories of problematic or harmful behaviors: Cognitive rigidity and an external locus of control (Morgan & Lilienfeld, 2000). Most directly, these might affect internal (and potentially external) capacity development in:

- Knowledge (For example, cognitive rigidity presents a barrier to learning, which involves thinking differently about subjects.)
- Relatedness (For example, an external locus of control can prevent taking effective action on one's responsibilities within a relationship.)
- Community (For example, rigidly believing that a community should exist within a particular structure and that other structures would be wrong. It might also include not seeing oneself as a participant in a community due to seeing only the community's impact on the client.)
- Inner peace (For example, a person may not believe that they can have peace unless their external circumstances change.)
- Creativity (For example, creativity often requires cognitive flexibility.)
- Agency (For example, not seeing oneself as capable of autonomy or independence due to an internal locus of control or rigid beliefs about one's circumstances.)
- Mastery at work (For example, rigidly believing that because one is subject to the whims of external circumstances, they cannot attain this PHG.)

Self-regulation. Clearly, it is difficult to be successful with any good life plan when one has problems with self-regulation. Without self-regulatory abilities, it is entirely possible that all PHGs can be directly affected, with some of the most pronounced effects occurring in:

- Life
- Mastery at work
- Mastery at play
- Agency
- Relatedness
- Community
- States of happiness and pleasure
- Inner peace

Ultimately, an awareness of the impact of trauma and adversity on PHG acquisition is fundamental to GLM practice.

A final note on multidisciplinary efforts in implementing the GLM with people who have histories of trauma and adversity is in order. The effects of early adversity on clients can touch every aspect of their lives. Implications for GLM practice include understanding that change for some clients may come slowly. After all, given the rates of issues with cognitive skills, such as rigid thinking and an external locus of control, no program or practitioner should expect that clients will be able to reassemble and improve their lives in a short period of time. A common message heard in inpatient programs using the GLM is the need for patience and understanding with clients.

4.13 The Role of Culture

The GLM cannot be properly implemented without respect for cultural differences between clients (Ward & Dickie, in press). While cultural awareness has been at the center of societal debates for centuries, a few points may be useful for GLM practice.

Practitioners should always keep in mind that culture can have a very different impact on clients. Therapists using the GLM may be viewed as state agents participating in systems of oppression. Even the ways that communities talk about culture can vary around the world; in some languages, the word "race" is not used because it is assumed that all people belong only to the human race.

PHGs are prioritized more in some cultures than others, and the impact of racism can present severe restrictions on external capacity (for example, through stigma, discrimination, and the lingering effects of colonization) and internal capacity (when racist beliefs become internalized). The question isn't whether the GLM works with clients of a given background, but rather, how the various cultures (including race, ethnicity, gender, sexuality, nationality, and religious background) in this person's life may have influenced their good life plan and how these can best be addressed within the GLM.

In some cases, applying the GLM will require knowledge of broad cultural aspects. As one example, the relationship of indigenous people to those descended from colonists can vary from one part of the world to another, requiring broad knowledge of the history in that region. In some instances, practitioners will have to focus on a more individualized basis (e.g., "our client came from an Eastern European country and is now here in our city. We are trying to learn from him what is important for us to know as we start GLM practice"). In one case, a conversation went along the lines of:

Client:	"I've heard about the GLM. It won't work for me."
Therapist:	"Why not?"
C:	"I'm Asian. The GLM is for white people."
T:	"I'm not sure I follow."
C:	"I've talked to the other guys here in the program. They keep talking about how their pursuit of 'agency' was all wrong and got them into trouble. They're out of the old cowboy movies! Everything they talk about has something to do with freedom and independence and autonomy and making their own decisions. I'm from an entirely different culture. For us, family is everything. Where I'm from if you ask me how I'm doing, I'd tell you about my family. If you ask me how I'm doing individually, I won't be able to answer as easily as those guys do."
T:	"Yes, those are some big differences. You're making some important points. Can I ask a couple of questions to see if I understand?"
C:	"Sure."
T:	"When you lived with your family, were there ever times you wanted to eat something different for dinner than what your mother was making?"
C:	"Yes, of course."
T:	"Did you ever dream of doing something for a living that might have been outside your family's plans for you?"
C:	"Definitely. I'm here, aren't I?"
T:	"Very true. Did you ever try to influence your family to do something that you wanted to do?"
C:	"Of course. What's your point?"
T:	"That developing agency can look very different in different cultures. Your family relationships really are important to you, yet they may not be everything. You may not be a lot like the others in the program, but you share a lot of things in common below the surface. What's different isn't your goals in life, but how important they are and how you go about making them happen. Does that make sense?"
C:	"Okay, I got it. And if I'd thought more about how those things work off each other, like making decisions about my actions, I might have prevented some big mistakes."
T (smiling):	"You've really been thinking about your life. Great work. It's not easy to put in that kind of effort."

With an understanding of the central themes in treatment and the role of seemingly thorny issues such as trauma, culture, and the role of the therapist, the rest of the chapter can focus on other practical considerations, including modalities, fidelity monitoring, and barriers to implementation.

4.14 GLM with Adolescents

It is worth noting here that the GLM is routinely adapted for use with adolescents (Fortune, 2018; Prescott, 2025; Print, 2013). It is noted throughout the available texts that applying the GLM to adolescents should never be a simple downward extension of methods for treating adults. Rather, much like approaches such as motivational interviewing (Miller & Rollnick, 2023), using the GLM with adolescents involves tailoring it to the unique characteristics of the client (see Chap. 5 for further discussion on emerging adults). The following overarching considerations are important:

- Professionals must understand the developmental aspects of the adolescent. Adolescents are typically in a state of constant change. Aspects such as decision-making, emotions, risk-taking, and sexuality are all typically still very much in development, requiring developmentally sensitive methods and approaches by adults.
- Professionals must also consider the environment in which the young person exists. Adolescents are, by definition, dependent upon the nature and quality of the contexts in which they find themselves.
- Professionals will need to keep in mind that the nature of internal and external capacities will change across adolescence, as will the other obstacles mentioned above. Further, their PHGs will also change, both with respect to importance (for example, seeing a stronger drive toward agency) and the means by which the young person seeks to attain them.

Finally, it is important to note that adolescents will naturally have less capacity to account fully for their actions, whether in the eyes of the law or in their therapists' offices. Readers are referred to other extant literature for applying the GLM to this age group.

4.15 GLM Modalities

As an overarching practice framework, the GLM lends itself to several modalities. It has been applied in case management (Purvis et al., 2013) as well as to therapeutic programs. It can be used in individual or group therapy.

Individual therapy. As a framework designed to be individualized, the GLM lends itself to individual therapy in a straightforward fashion. Elsewhere in this volume, the GLM mapping tool and intervention plan can help to guide treatment. Individual therapy also lends itself to more extensive conversations on topics that a client may be reluctant to bring up in group.

Group therapy. There is a rich literature on group therapy in forensic contexts (e.g., Sawyer & Jennings, 2016) leaving no doubt as to its potential for helping clients to build better lives for themselves. Depending on circumstances, group therapists might consider conducting groups in an open fashion, with each client discussing various aspects of the GLM that they are working on and getting feedback from others. Those who are further along in treatment can ask questions and provide support to those who are newer, and all members can review their efforts at developing skills and other forms of capacities. Another option can be for the therapist(s) to develop exercises based on GLM principles, such as how clients are working to develop capacities with respect to a good life goal. There are many possibilities (for example, the use of music in Chap. 6).

One option for group therapy can be to use a workbook exercise as the start of a discussion topic for the session (e.g., Prescott, 2025; Prescott & Dent, 2016; Prescott & Pflugradt, 2024; Prescott et al., 2023). In some settings, the clients may begin group by quickly reviewing an exercise in the workbook that they completed on their own time, reading their answers out loud to the group, after which the facilitator starts a discussion and clients offer feedback to one another. This approach has been helpful in settings with clients whose special needs may make group participation challenging (and who presumably are also receiving individual therapy). Under no conditions should the workbook be mistaken for a prescribed curriculum, but rather as a tool for clinical discussion.

In some high-intensity inpatient programs, the therapist may give the paraprofessional staff exercises to use with clients that focus on PHG acquisition. These non-clinical topics might involve skills for getting and maintaining a job (mastery at work); independent living skills (life); relaxation (inner peace); skills for community activities to prevent awkward, uncomfortable, or even illegal interactions with others (community); and the like. Some programs display artwork on the walls with GLM themes that can help with these discussions. One program had the clients paint one wall of their common area with a picture of a tree; each branch was named after a PHG.

The one caution in any application of the GLM practice framework is ensuring that a clinical specialist with the appropriate degree and license/registration oversees the activities to ensure that the style, spirit, vision, and technical aspects of the GLM are followed correctly.

4.16 Fidelity Monitoring

Helping programs and practitioners to maintain fidelity to the GLM has been a major focus of recent efforts and resulted in a tool that is widely available in English, French, and Dutch (Prescott et al., 2022a, 2022b; Prescott & Willis, 2021a; Ward et al., 2024). It covers three areas: Fundamental considerations and processes, GLM-specific considerations and processes, and client-focused GLM considerations. The tool has scoring instructions and ideas for its best use, primarily as a tool for consultation, supervision, and self-reflection.

Fundamental Considerations and Processes This section includes a focus on the qualities of the therapist as perceived by the client and others, a review of the underlying spirit of treatment delivery, how the therapist prioritizes clinical skills that promote change, and actively and explicitly seeking client feedback.

GLM-Specific Considerations and Processes This examines the extent to which the therapist focuses on the PHGs generally and those PHGs implicated in harmful behaviors, conceptualizes risk factors, and focuses on activities that ameliorate the obstacles to one's good life plan.

Client-Focused GLM Considerations This consists of 10 questions exploring therapists' progress developing a GLM-grounded case conceptualization and therapy plan for individual clients.

Even the best of therapists can sometimes drift off course or develop habits and practices that do not entirely comport with the GLM. With the proliferation of programs seeking to implement the GLM comes the need to consider many perspectives on its successful application. At a minimum, the GLM Fidelity Monitoring Tool enables users to examine their alignment with broader elements of the GLM as well as the processes within it (Prescott et al., 2022a, 2022b).

4.17 GLM Implementation

The GLM has been implemented in diverse settings and circumstances in many areas around the world. Over time, research has emerged to guide programs in how to implement new programs and what challenges one might expect (Brattland et al., 2018; Fixsen et al., 2005). In our experience, there are several beliefs held by programs and practitioners that can impede meaningful implementation (Prescott & Willis, 2021b). These include:

Lack of Support by Leadership Applying the GLM requires that programs and practitioners possess certain attributes and engage in processes often referred to as a program's "culture." As with any workplace or educational setting, if the people who oversee the program are not invested in the GLM, it is less likely to be implemented well. When considering GLM implementation, ensuring leadership buy-in is often the most important first task.

The Belief That "we already do this" It can be easy for those who first encounter the GLM to form premature judgments about it. Often this takes the form of seeing its commonalities to other forms of psychotherapy (for example, the importance of the therapeutic alliance) and assuming that it must be like those methods with which the practitioner is already familiar. In some cases, this belief can result in confirmation bias, whereby the individual disregards aspects of the GLM with which they are not familiar or believe that since they have the general idea, they have enough information to stop their learning. As described elsewhere (Prescott & Willis, 2021b), questions for new GLM practitioners to consider include:

- Is the practitioner using the actual PHGs described in the GLM?
- Is the practitioner using the PHGs as they are defined? The PHGs as constructed have an empirical foundation described in the foundational writings (e.g., Ward & Stewart, 2003; Yates et al., 2010).
- Can the practitioner identify which PHGs are important to this client?
- Has the practitioner explored the client's practical identity?
- Can the practitioner describe how the PHGs were implicated (or not implicated) in the client's problematic behaviors?
- Does the practitioner have a solid understanding of how PHGs interact with causal processes implicated in the client's offending?
- Has the practitioner conducted a solid assessment of the client's strengths (as they relate to prosocial acquisition of PHGs) and accounted for how the client can apply them to treatment and to his or her life beyond treatment more effectively?
- Has the practitioner explored the vertical and horizontal coherence of the client's good life plan?
- Can the practitioner identify the obstacles in the client's good life plan?
- Can the practitioner identify how the client has sought to implement a good life plan in the past, in the present, and how they plan to implement in the future?
- Have the practitioner and client arrived at the answers to questions such as how the client and others around them will know that they are attaining a good effectively or ineffectively?

The Belief That "this is easy" Learning portions of the GLM or learning about it is not the same as developing deep practice expertise. High-quality implementation takes time, effort, and practice; this fact is in line with the findings of implementation research with many models. Ultimately, study, training, and supervision/consultation are all vital in putting the GLM into practice.

Simplifying the GLM The authors have been aware of occasional attempts to simplify the GLM, often by removing PHGs and related goals that the therapist, administration, or researcher deems to be superfluous, such as spirituality or states of happiness and pleasure. Often these decisions have been made without consultation with the clients they serve. Such simplifications can become reductionistic and contrary to the holistic underpinnings of the GLM. Similar simplification can occur when personal opinions interfere with implementation. One colleague who was unfamiliar with the GLM stated that, "It's time we go beyond the GLM and use mindfulness as the centerpiece of our program." This person had been unaware of the PHGs of inner peace and spirituality at the time. Different clients will need shorter and longer lengths of treatment but altering the GLM to speed up treatment or slow it down will not improve outcomes in the long run.

4.18 Conclusion

Applying the GLM in therapy and treatment programs requires patience and commitment, but its holistic nature typically means a more impactful experience for the client. Its nature as a practice framework is often a new experience for those who have been trained primarily in specific protocols. Its implementation across programs often involves training, supervision, consultation, and practitioner self-reflection. The case examples included in Chap. 8 may contribute to a sense of how best to apply the model in different circumstances.

References

Beech, A. R., & Fordham, A. S. (1997). Therapeutic climate of sexual offender treatment programs. *Sexual Abuse: A Journal of Research and Treatment, 9*, 219–237.

Brattland, H., Koksvik, J. M., Burkeland, O., Gråwe, R. W., Klöckner, C., Linaker, O. M., Ryum, T., Wampold, B., Lara-Cabrera, M. L., & Iversen, V. C. (2018). The effects of routine outcome monitoring (ROM) on therapy outcomes in the course of an implementation process: A randomized clinical trial. *Journal of Counseling Psychology, 65*(5), 641–652. https://doi.org/10.1037/cou0000286

Bordin, E. S. (1979). The generalizability of the psychoanalytic concept of the working alliance. *Psychotherapy: Theory Research & Practice, 16*, 252–260.

Chow, D. (2017). The practice and the practical: Pushing your clinical performance to the next level. In D. S. Prescott, C. L. Maeschalck, & S. D. Miller (Eds.), *Feedback-informed treatment in clinical practice: Reaching for excellence* (pp. 323–355). American Psychological Association. https://doi.org/10.1037/0000039-017

Drapeau, M. (2005). Research on the processes involved in treating sexual offenders. *Sexual Abuse: A Journal of Research and Treatment, 17*, 117–125.

Fixsen, D., Naoom, S., Blase, K., Friedman, R., & Wallace, F. (2005). *Implementation research: A synthesis of the literature*. University of South Florida, Louis de la Parte Florida Mental Health Institute, National Implementation Research Network.

Fortune, C.-A. (2018). The good lives model: A strength-based approach for youth offenders. *Aggression and Violent Behavior, 38*, 21–30. https://doi.org/10.1016/j.avb.2017.11.003

Glaser, B. (2011). Paternalism and the good lives model of sex offender rehabilitation. *Sexual abuse: a journal of research and treatment, 23*(3), 329–345. https://doi.org/10.1177/1079063210382044

Levenson, J. S., Grady, M. D., Lasoski, H., & Collins, K. T. (2024). Learning from consumers of mandated sex-offending programs: "It's not Treatment, I wish it was". *Sexual Abuse, 36*(2), 203–232. https://doi.org/10.1177/10790632231172158

Levenson, J. S., & Willis, G. M. (2019). Implementing trauma-informed care in correctional treatment and supervision. *Journal of Aggression, Maltreatment & Trauma, 28*(4), 481–501. https://doi.org/10.1080/10926771.2018.1531959

Levenson, J. S., Willis, G., & Prescott, D. (2017). *Trauma-informed care: Transforming treatment for people who sexually abuse*. Safer Society Press.

Linehan, M. M. (2014). *DBT (R) skills training handouts and worksheets* (2nd ed.). Guilford Publications.

Marshall, W. L. (2005). Therapist style in sexual offender treatment: Influence on indices of change. *Sexual Abuse: Journal of Research and Treatment, 17*(2), 109–116. https://doi.org/10.1177/107906320501700202

Miller, W. R., & Rollnick, S. (2023). *Motivational interviewing: Helping people change and grow* (4th ed.). The Guilford Press, A Division of Guilford Publications, Inc.
Morgan, A. B., & Lilienfeld, S. O. (2000). A meta-analytic review of the relation between antisocial behavior and neuropsychological measures of executive function. *Clinical Psychology Review, 20*(1), 113–136. https://doi.org/10.1016/s0272-7358(98)00096-8[1]
Norcross, J. C. (2010). The therapeutic relationship. In B. L. Duncan, S. D. Miller, B. E. Wampold, & M. A. Hubble (Eds.), *The heart and soul of change: Delivering what works in therapy* (2nd ed., pp. 113–141). American Psychological Association.
Parhar, K. K., Wormith, J. S., Derkzen, D. M., & Beauregard, A. M. (2008). Offender coercion in treatment: A metaanalysis of effectiveness. *Criminal Justice and Behavior, 35*(9), 1109–1135.
Prescott, D. S., Maeschalck, C. L., & Miller, S. D. (Eds.). (2017). *Feedback-informed treatment in clinical practice: Reaching for excellence*. American Psychological Association.
Prescott, D. S., Maeschalck, C. M., & Miller, S. D. (2022a). Feedback-informed treatment. In R. Fulmer (Ed.), *Counseling and psychotherapy: Theory and beyond*. Cognella.
Prescott, D. S., Willis, G. M., & Ward, T. (2022b). Monitoring therapist fidelity to the good lives model (GLM). *International Journal of Offender Therapy and Comparative Criminology*. https://doi.org/10.1177/0306624X221086572
Prescott, D. S. (2025). *Becoming who I want to be: A good lives workbook* (2nd ed.). Safer Society Press.
Prescott, D. S., & Dent, T. (2016). *Becoming who I want to be: A good lives workbook for young women*. Safer Society Press.
Prescott, D. S., & Pflugradt, D. (2024). *Becoming the man I want to be: A good lives workbook* (2nd ed.). Safer Society Press.
Prescott, D. S., Pflugradt, D. M., & Allen, B. P. (2023). *Becoming the woman I want to be: A good lives workbook*. Safer Society Press.
Prescott, D. S., & Willis, G. M. (2021a). Evaluation de la fidélité des professionnels au Good Lives Model (GLM). In E. Dieu, E. Zinsstag, & T. Ward (Eds.), *Special Issue "Criminologie de la confiance et Good Lives Model (GLM)"*. Revue Internationale de Criminologie et de Police Technique et Scientifique.
Prescott, D. S., & Willis, G. M. (2021b). Using the good lives model (GLM) in clinical practice: Lessons learned from international implementations. *Aggression and Violent Behavior*. https://doi.org/10.1016/j.avb.2021.101717
Print, B. (Ed.). (2013). *The good lives model for adolescents who sexually harm*. Safer Society Press.
Purvis, M., Ward, T., & Shaw, S. (2013). *Applying the good lives model to the case management of sexual offenders*. Safer Society Press.
Ross, E., Polaschek, D., & Ward, T. (2008). The therapeutic alliance: A theoretical revision for offender rehabilitation. *Aggression and Violent Behavior, 13*, 462–480.
Sawyer, S., & Jennings, J. L. (2016). *Group therapy with sexual abusers: Engaging the full potential of the group experience*. Safer Society Press.
Shapiro, F. (2018). *Eye movement desensitization and reprocessing (EMDR) therapy: Basic principles, protocols, and procedures* (3rd ed.). Guilford Press.
Ward, T. & Dickie, I. (in press). An enactive conception of sexual offending: Integrating biological, psychological, and cultural factors. In I. Dickie, S. Wareham, & A Beech (Eds.), Cultural responsivity issues: Treatment of sexual. : Routledge.
Ward, T., & Stewart, C. A. (2003). The treatment of sex offenders: Risk management and good lives. *Professional Psychology: Research and Practice, 34*, 353–360. https://doi.org/10.1037/0735-7028.34.4.353
Ward, T., Willis, G. M., & Prescott, D. S. (2024). The rehabilitation of corrections clients: Good lives and risk reduction. In G. M. Davies & A. R. Beech (Eds.), *Forensic psychology: Crime, justice, law, interventions* (pp. 511–531). Wiley.
Walfish, S., McAlister, B., O'Donnell, P., & Lambert, M. J. (2012). An investigation of self-assessment bias in mental health providers. *Psychological Reports, 110*(2), 1–6. https://doi.org/10.2466/02.07.17.PR0.110.2.2
Yates, P., Prescott, D., & Ward, T. (2010). *Applying the good lives and self regulation models to sex offender treatment: A practical guide for clinicians*. Safer Society Press.

Chapter 5
Reentry Issues and Interventions

5.1 Introduction

This chapter concerns the challenges facing people who have lived, often for many years, in prisons, psychiatric institutions, and various residential settings as they move closer to reentering the community. It explores the changes in practical identity that can take place and the role that both intrinsic and extrinsic motivations can play in the lives of those clients reentering the community. It reviews the role of case managers and probation agents, highlights the experiences of emerging adults, and offers examples of GLM implementation at system-wide levels. Critical to providing the GLM framework to individuals who are reentering or moving closer to the community is appreciating how many changes are involved in adjusting to the challenges of desistance (see Chap. 1).

5.2 Background

The failure of coercive approaches and imprisonment to reduce recidivism or to help people lead more effective lives is well established in the research literature (Aos et al., 2006; Parhar et al., 2008; Petrich et al., 2021; Smith et al., 2002). A review by Petrich et al. (2021) in this regard is noteworthy and can help guide practitioners using the GLM. Petrich et al. (2021) describe the extant research succinctly:

> Based on past research and the findings of this meta-analysis, the limited effects of custodial sanctions on reoffending should be viewed as a criminological fact… The highest quality studies reduce the criminogenic effect of custodial sanctions but do not eliminate it. This meta-analysis of a large sample of heterogeneous studies reaches the same conclusion. Narrative reviews do also. Consensus that custodial sanctions, overall, do not reduce reoffending is universal (p. 41).

T. Ward et al., *The Good Lives Model of Correctional Rehabilitation*,
Advances in Preventing and Treating Violence and Aggression,
https://doi.org/10.1007/978-3-031-95559-4_5

In some cases, the situation can be even more dire. A recent study by Fitch et al. (2024) found that the rate of suicide among people following incarceration was double that of the general population for 3 years after release, and at its highest in the 2 weeks immediately following release. Emerging adults were among those at elevated risk. These results provide some of the unfortunate background for many clients entering treatment using the GLM. Paying closer attention to clients' personal priorities and associated practical identities is likely to result in better social and psychological outcomes than simply focusing on risk reduction.

Criminological and desistance research can help to illustrate the ways forward with clients. At a practical level, however, a question remains: While we often talk about community reentry and reintegration, how many of our clients were ever actually fully integrated in their communities to begin with? Is "reintegration" a misnomer? Perhaps "integration" is the more proper term in many cases. Understanding that many of our clients will be attempting reentry into a community that they may never have been a part of can sometimes be the most helpful place to start in applying the GLM following incarceration (McCartan et al., 2018). As a result, this chapter uses the term "reentry" with the understanding that clients often have a long history of viewing themselves, and being viewed, as moral strangers—that is, as deeply flawed, unfathomable, and "contaminated" individuals who are best managed at arm's length, and kept isolated from the rest of the community in order to keep everyone else safe from harm.

5.3 Changes in Practical Identity

GLM interventions center on a personally meaningful good life plan, containing all primary goods to varying degrees (chosen by the individual), and the secondary goods (goals and strategies) required to attain these without harming others (Willis et al., 2024). This can be linked with risk reduction by identifying the goods sought via offending (either directly or indirectly) in the past and the barriers or problems (i.e., criminogenic needs) evident within the strategies used to attain these goods. For example, sexual offending might have been used to achieve relatedness or pleasure because of problems differentiating between appropriate partners (i.e., children are preferred as sexual partners because individuals feel emotionally safer with them). A new good life plan (GLP) could incorporate relatedness and pleasure via the goal of seeking an intimate relationship with an age-appropriate consenting partner. Strategies may include attending social activities, creating an online dating profile, engaging in conversation, physical intimacy, vulnerable disclosure, conflict resolution, and so on. Individuals vary in their ability to engage in these normative practices; the capacities required for healthy intimacy are learned and shaped via social interaction. Therapy can target risk factors such as emotional congruence with children through the development or strengthening of internal and external capacities and resources. This might include developing healthy beliefs about the self, others, and relationships (e.g., "others are trustworthy," "I am safe"), communication and negotiation skills, emotion management, perspective-taking, and so on. In addition, the availability of external resources (e.g., opportunity, finances, freedom) can support or obstruct goods attainment and should be included in a GLP. Essentially, an intervention plan should identify the most heavily weighted goods (which are linked to a person's practical identity and sense of meaning) and those sought via offending, use these to construct a comprehensive GLP, and then develop or strengthen the internal and external resources required to live a good life without reoffending. The GLM proposes a dual focus on promoting goods and overcoming barriers (i.e., problems signaled by DRFs), it does this in collaboration with the individual to build on strengths and focus on meaningful personal goals, rather than simply avoiding reoffending.

As professionals begin to consider applying the GLM to individuals, whether before or after their transition from a more structured situation to a less structured setting, these clients are virtually always undergoing profound changes to their practical identity (see Chaps. 1 and 8). By this we mean self-descriptions under which individuals find core features of themselves and their lives of value. For example:

John spent 10 years in the psychiatric wing of a prison following convictions on charges related to selling drugs, possessing illegal weapons, and assaulting one of the officers who arrested him. He was released to a community-based residential program with another several years of probation. While in prison, his single most prioritized PHGs were life and agency. As he recounted in his assessment interview in the program, the entire decade of his incarceration was spent trying to survive the hostile and traumagenic environment of a psychiatric prison (PHG of life). Within this experience, he also tried to maintain as much of his independence and autonomy (agency) as he could. Given that he had no choice over who he shared a cell with, what he ate, what hours he kept, or even who was on his treatment and case management teams, he cherished every opportunity he had to make decisions for himself.

With his focus on life and agency, he had very little external capacity for achieving the other PHGs, although he was starting to think about what options would be available. In his own words describing the other PHGs:

Mastery at work. "I had a job cleaning the kitchen and cafeteria. Toward the end, they let me load supplies off a truck into the kitchen. Now that I'm here, I hope I can do something like that and someday maybe get some kind of job in the community."

Mastery at play. "They let me go to the gym and get some exercise. Mostly I walked around the gym. A lot of the guys played basketball, but I didn't really fit in, and it sometimes got kind of rough. I didn't want any trouble. I see they have more activities here; maybe I can try some of those. I was hoping I could have a typewriter and practice writing things."

Community. "There was a lot of things going on that weren't supposed to happen, so I kept to myself as much as possible. I don't know if anyone even remembers me in the town that I'm from, and I'm probably not allowed to go there. I could ask my probation officer, but it's better if I don't go back. I'm just happy to be right here where I am. I guess I'm not cut out for community living. Maybe someday. The one thing I really want to do is attend NA (Narcotics Anonymous) meetings in the community."

Knowledge. "I got some drug counseling in prison, and I learned a lot about that. They really helped me. Also, I took some classes when I was inside. I learned a bit about math and learned more about how to read. I guess mostly I learned how to follow orders and not talk back. I guess I'm grateful for that. I really learned how to not say what was on my mind. It kept me out of a lot of trouble. Now that I'm here, I would love to take some kind of class. I don't know what I'm allowed to do."

Relatedness. "I used to talk to the psychologist. That guy helped me a lot. Mostly he listened and he taught me some skills for getting along. I haven't heard from my family since before I was arrested. I don't know where they are. In prison I kept to myself. Now that I'm here, I hope I get along with the others. My big dream would be to meet someone and maybe have a family, but that's a long way off and it's better if I just focus on myself for now."

States of happiness and pleasure. "I used some drugs my first year in prison, but it got to be too much. I've noticed they show movies down in the living room here, and I like that."

Creativity. "I like to draw sometimes. I took an art class in prison. I used to have a guitar before I got arrested. Prison life doesn't allow for a lot of new experiences, but I'm willing to try."

Spirituality. "I took a Bible study correspondence course in prison. I read sections of the Bible—with some help from the chaplain—and answered questions on a worksheet. Sometimes I went to the services at the chapel in prison. I'd like to do more of that. Honestly, I haven't been able to think about this all very much, but I do really want to. As for where I fit into the universe… Honestly, I don't know, but I'm grateful for the opportunity to be here in this program. I am really grateful."

Inner peace. "I think I told you. I didn't really have any peace in prison; there were gangs and kids fighting all the time. I learned to meditate, and I tried that. I'm not very good at it, but the teacher told me everyone says that. Now that I'm here, I like watching the leaves on the trees outside my window, especially when they blow in the breeze. That's like peace."

In assessing John's implicit GLP at the time of his discharge (he did not receive GLM treatment in the prison), it becomes clear that community reentry will not be easy. The restrictions placed on him in the psychiatric prison have acted as a source of reduced external capacity to acquire the PHGs but have compelled John to pursue a very different lifestyle within the institution; one marked by an almost entirely external locus of control. Against that backdrop, John's opportunities to develop internal capacity—that is, the skills he needs for PHG acquisition—are virtually non-existent. Furthermore, whatever internal capacity he did develop in the psychiatric prison would not translate well into community living. A final challenge is that the survival-oriented lifestyle that clients develop in prison and similar institutions is often very narrow in scope.

It is, therefore, no surprise that John's GLP as he reentered the community lacks vertical coherence. His survival meant focusing on life and agency with little time to focus on the other PHGs. Likewise, his GLP lacked horizontal coherence. With few opportunities to develop his internal capacities to attain the other PHGs, his GLP is poorly integrated, and he is unprepared for the challenges that lie ahead.

A study by Harris et al. (2019) found that John's experience is common. The two most important PHGs for people reentering the community are *life* and *relatedness*. Within John's description above are indications that, now that he has been released, he hopes 1 day to be more connected to others. In a broader perspective, however, the work of Harris et al. (2019) and John's case both point to how community reentry can be a time of turmoil for individuals, one in which dramatic changes to one's PHG are to be expected. At the very least, clients like John can expect:

- Changes in practical identity
- Changes in vertical and horizontal coherence
- Unforeseen changes in external capacity to work towards PHG acquisition
- Re-assessment of their internal capacity to achieve goals related to PHGs
- Upheaval in the importance of PHGs previously not prioritized

5.4 Intrinsic and Extrinsic Motivations

In their work on self-determination theory, Ryan and Deci (2000, 2017) describe two types of motivation that are relevant to reentry and the GLM: intrinsic (undertaking an activity for its own sake rather than for an external benefit) and extrinsic (an external catalyst for taking an action). A complete description of self-determination theory is beyond the scope of this chapter, but aspects of it can illustrate some of the challenges faced in reentry. In the broadest sense, many mandated clients enter treatment because of extrinsic factors (it's often a condition of release), and eventually become more intrinsically motivated to make lasting, positive changes to their life. Within the broader category of extrinsic motivation, Ryan & Deci distinguish four types, including:

- *Purely external motivation* (seeking a reward or avoiding a consequence)
- *Introjected motivation* (a mostly external state involving efforts at active self-control)
- *Identified motivation* (a mostly internal state in which actions reflect conscious decisions and personal values)
- *Integrated motivation* (an internal state in which actions reflect congruence with one's values)

When working with reentry issues, it can be useful to keep these motivations in mind. While the PHGs that clients in therapy pursue are intrinsically motivating, the tasks to achieve them may be more complicated. For example, in the case described above, when John was making the transition from psychiatric prison to the residential program in the community, he could expect to experience several forms of extrinsic motivation. The fact remained that he would be under strict supervision by a probation officer for several years (external motivation). He would initially participate in group treatment out of introjected motivation. That is, his initial response to group therapy was that he did not want to attend it but recognized that it was an expectation of his placement, and he did not want to cause anyone to contact his probation officer or consider returning him to prison. He happily participated in individual therapy sessions out of identified motivation because he enjoyed feeling heard, understood, and respected and knew that each session served to help him acquire the PHGs in the long term.

There are several reasons why reviewing these activities and motivations with clients can be useful to promoting the most effective therapeutic outcomes:

Exploring and resolving ambivalence. Beginning a treatment program can often be more challenging to clients than it seems. The therapist and client can review client ambivalence about the tasks of treatment that are aimed at overcoming obstacles to the client's PHG acquisition. For example, while group therapy can be a highly rewarding experience that brings about lasting change, clients are often ambivalent about entering a group. Insight into the nature of the client's motivations and ambivalence can help the client shift their motivation for participation into a more internal direction.

Eliciting client feedback. Being aware of the changing nature of client motivation can help therapists and other professionals to tailor services throughout the course of treatment.

Refocusing and returning to the PHGs. A client's focus in treatment may vary over time. The promise, allure, and intrinsically motivating nature of the PHGs can sometimes get lost in the client's mind when they are focused on the daily tasks of life in their community reentry efforts. In the case of John, the intrinsic motivation of examining the PHGs would quickly erode at those times when his motivation for some aspects of change (such as medication compliance or regular attendance in group therapy) would wane.

An example from outside of GLM application may also illustrate the importance of attending to these motivations. Sheldon (2020) studied the motivations of long-distance hikers. He found that those who completed the 2650-mile (4270 km) Pacific Coast Trail in the USA often started with intrinsic motivation; the time spent on the trail was its own reward. As the hikers continued, often through grueling conditions, their motivations changed to *identified*. This means that they continued to hike through often challenging conditions because continuing was in line with their values. Recast in the language of PHGs, they began their hike aspiring to agency, life, mastery at play, inner peace, and states of happiness and pleasure. They continued onward aspiring to spirituality (their persistence providing a sense of meaning and purpose).

To summarize up to this point:

- Community reentry can be challenging in situations where the client has never entirely been a part of the community they came from.
- Apart from the treatment programs that may exist in their walls, prisons and similar institutions do not reduce risk for re-offense.
- The first weeks and months following release from prisons and similar institutions are a time of intense vulnerability for clients.
- The importance of PHGs in each client's GLP can change, often dramatically. This means that their practical identities are also subject to change unless *vertical coherence* can be created, that is, links established between prioritized PHGs, secondary goods, and their associated daily practices.
- There are significant differences in the obstacles for achieving PHGs as one reenters the community. For example, there are significant changes to internal and external capacity demands, such as unanticipated social demand for which the person lacks adaptive responses. A client may have had a very narrow scope to their GLP while in the institution.
- Motivation to change, like motivation to participate in treatment, can fluctuate over time and is important to assess regularly. Some aspects of the reentry process will be subject to different forms of motivation, and addressing these can be important to treatment outcomes.

5.5 Barriers to Therapy in Reentry

As if the changing nature of practical identities,[1] motivation, and internal/external capacity weren't enough, there are other barriers to reentry worthy of discussion. The barriers discussed below are not exhaustive but are worthy of consideration when helping clients make the transition out of institutions.

Post-conviction traumatic stress. In the USA, Harris and Levenson (2020) studied the reentry experience of people who have often experienced traumatic stress in prison and then return to traumagenic experiences in the community. They conceptualized their findings as post-conviction traumatic stress and took note that many who reenter the community are not able to meet their basic human needs. Further, this inability to meet their needs interfered with their efforts at desisting from further crime (as predicted by GLM knowledge assumptions; see Chap. 1). They concluded that, as it is constructed, the criminal justice system itself is traumagenic. In the past, this stress has been easy for professionals to overlook, in part because incarceration followed the client's actions. It is easy to forget the

[1] Practical identities tend to be stable once acquired but can be destabilized by unexpected personal and social demands. This is in part because they are relatively new and because environmental challenges can be more or less reinforcing of newly formed self-conceptions. For example, someone who recently adopted a new practical identity of loving father and partner may find this self-description difficult to maintain when faced with unrelenting social criticism and rejection, and financial hardship. That is, when there is a lack of vertical and horizontal coherency.

high levels of traumatic stress that clients often bring with them into treatment (Levenson et al., 2017). Screening for this in clinical interviews is therefore advisable.

Labels. The ethics of labeling has been discussed at length in the literature and in this volume (see Chap. 10). As Willis (2018) has noted, the labels applied to clients (such as felon, registrant, mentally ill, etc.) can interfere with efforts at desistance, self-efficacy, and cognitive transformation (Maruna et al., 2004). These considerations are very important for professionals to remember when working with correctional clients and are in line with similar dialogues in the mental health field (for example, the American Psychological Association's [APA] move toward inclusive language; APA, 2023). However, an awareness of the effects of labels at the individual level is also critical for successful reentry.

To illustrate this effect of labels, consider this statement from the introduction to an assessment report: "Mr. X is a 28-year-old gay Black male found incompetent to stand trial on charges of first-degree sexual assault. In his most recent psychiatric hospitalization, he was diagnosed with schizoaffective disorder, autism spectrum disorder, and personality disorder not otherwise specified." Reading this statement at the start of an intake process for treatment poses a high risk of activating biases in the reader, many of which may be beyond their awareness. Unless the client prefers it mentioned at the start of the report, is it necessary to state from the outset that someone is gay unless there is a compelling reason to do so? Is it necessary to reference their race?

While sharing legal and diagnostic information is certainly an important part of the process, it is also important to be sensitive to the implicit and explicit biases that may alter the course of subsequent assessment and treatment efforts. These sentences would have been more effective had they been rewritten in a way that assists the reader in designing interventions. Whatever the case, professionals using the GLM will wish to remain on guard for the biasing effects of labels, which may distract from the full range of potential interventions. Because many clients leaving institutions often have complicated clinical presentations, this awareness of bias is all the more important.

A more GLM-adherent way to write the sentences above might be:

Mr. X is 28 years old. He has faced many challenges in recent years. After being abandoned by his family in his teenage years, he spent time in homeless shelters and was eventually hospitalized. Mr. X has faced considerable challenges involving developmental disabilities, which have limited his internal and external capacities for meeting his needs. These diagnoses include schizoaffective disorder, autism spectrum disorder, and personality disorder not otherwise specified. Mr. X has also experienced problems being accepted in his community (he is gay) and often experienced racism (he is Black). Most recently, he was charged with first-degree sexual assault stemming from an incident in which he attempted to force a man in his apartment building to have sex with him. He was of the belief that he was entering a relationship with this man. The man expressed that this was not the case.

Institutional syndrome (sometimes known as becoming institutionalized). Professionals treating clients who have spent long periods of time in institutions observe that these individuals often emerge with a dearth of skills for independent living and socializing with others. Institutional syndrome has sometimes been likened to a form of "slow death" due to the long-term effects of anxiety on physical health (Crane, 2019). The deprivation of independence and autonomy that can occur directly impacts their pursuit of agency. It is not uncommon to hear in these clients' statements an external locus of control; that is, that the events of their life unfold by chance or as a result of circumstances and others' actions. Not surprisingly, the resulting lack of self-efficacy can impede therapeutic progress, often with clients seeming to ask simply to be told what to do in order to complete therapy. In some cases, they may not seem to have any long-term plans or sense of meaning and purpose (PHG of spirituality) in their lives.

When therapists face clients with institutional syndrome, it can be important to return to the basics of the GLM, which proposes that all human beings are naturally motivated to seek the PHGs. There may be several reasons that a given client has institutional syndrome, including that it is a response to earlier life adversity or an adaptation to years spent in settings that restrict agency. In some cases, medical conditions also contribute to the broader sense of helplessness and loss of autonomy. Often, the client has simply given up hope. While therapists will need to be patient when dealing with institutional syndrome, a few ideas include:

- Exploring the client's ambivalence around efforts at making changes to his life.
- Reflectively listening to their thoughts about making meaningful changes to their life.
- Listening and reflecting back how the client's statements may link to the PHGs. For example, low motivation to change may be linked to inner peace by the client's hope that by not participating meaningfully in treatment they will remain free from the emotional turmoil it brings.
- Exploring, affirming, and validating positive changes that the client has made in the past, no matter how small they might be.
- Exploring the smallest differences with respect to where the client is in their lives and where they would like to be within a few months' (or weeks) time.
- Understanding and conveying to other professionals that while it took many years for the client to find themselves in these circumstances, it will likely take some time for them to find their way back out.
- Reframing for others that passive participation in treatment may also be a response (however maladaptive) to circumstances that erode personal agency.
- *Diagnosed and undiagnosed brain injuries*. Harmon (2012) has observed that people who are incarcerated in the USA have rates of brain injury that are seven times higher than the general population. By Harmon's reckoning, approximately 60% of incarcerated people have experienced one traumatic brain injury. Such injuries can result in problems with behavior (e.g., lack of persistence at tasks), emotions (e.g., irritability), impulsivity (e.g., engaging in high-risk behaviors), cognitive (e.g., impaired attentional processes), and other effects. As one

might expect, these are the same consequences that can interfere with treatment engagement, lead to longer periods of incarceration and similar placements, and result in further arrests. Sadly, this condition often goes unrecognized and misunderstood in treatment programs, especially those that do not take a holistic view of their clients. The implications of brain injury for assessment, treatment, and community reentry are serious and yet receive very little empirical attention. Perhaps the single most important implication for GLM practitioners is the need to clarify for others that problematic behaviors on the part of these clients may not be due to the client simply choosing to do so. That is, their ability to exercise responsible and effective agency is impaired in some respect.

- *Fetal Alcohol Syndrome Disorders (FASD).* Little is known about the rates of fetal alcohol syndrome among incarcerated individuals. Popova et al. (2011) estimated that in any given year, Canadian youth with FASD diagnoses were 19 times more likely to be incarcerated than youths without it. The authors noted that little data in this area is available outside of North America. As with traumatic brain injuries, the symptoms can often be masked as volitional behaviors when, in fact, they are medically based; that is, they are beyond a person's control. Difficulties concentrating, retaining information, impulsivity, and hyperactivity are all potential consequences of FASD. Practitioners using the GLM are advised to reframe these issues as medically based internal obstacles to the attainment of PHGs for other professionals and paraprofessionals who may view these symptoms from a purely behavioral perspective.

5.6 Case Management and Probation

Reentry to the community can be a time of great vulnerability in the life of a client. It can be essential to involve supervising agents such as case managers and probation officers as supports in assessment, planning, and treatment (Purvis et al., 2013). Typically, the role of case managers and probation officers involves such tasks as gathering information, carrying out court orders, and supporting efforts at rehabilitation. This last role is of fundamental importance. It can be easy to downplay the role of paraprofessionals in helping clients who have never experienced support in their communities before. Within probation settings, research has demonstrated that the relationship between client and officer can be a matter of public safety (Blasko et al., 2015). Likewise, intervention methods such as Circles of Support and Accountability that enlist professionally supervised volunteers to provide support can achieve dramatically improved outcomes (Wilson et al., 2009). GLM practitioners are therefore urged to use these resources to the best of their abilities whenever possible. Reentering a community means forming relationships with others who live there, and these professionals are sometimes the first people with whom clients can form a bond.

5.7 Emerging Adults

All too often, adults who reenter the community were originally removed from it as children or adolescents. These cases can often pose special challenges for professionals. For example, the nature of their long-term out-of-home placements may have left them with the institutional syndrome described above. Individuals' emerging agency may have been severely restricted, resulting in a lack of both internal and external capacity. Because they focused on a narrower range of life activities than their peers in the community, they may often have a narrow scope to their GLP prior to entering GLM therapy. They are more likely to have experienced the medical problems noted above and thus be more difficult to engage and appear less motivated for treatment. From the outside, they may appear not to understand that they have entered the world of adulthood, where agency and an internal locus of control are not only prized, but necessary for competent and adaptive functioning. From the inside, they are now living in a world that they have dreamed of but do not understand. The survival-based modes of interacting with others learned in adolescent programs no longer apply as they try to develop real-world adult-living skills in a short window of time. A case example may be helpful in illustrating some of the challenges of implementing the GLM with emerging adults:

5.7.1 Jack

Jack was 13 when he stole his mother's car, ran away from home, and wrecked the vehicle several miles away. He recalls his motivation for this as being a cry for help but would sometimes describe it as an overt act of revenge toward his brothers. Jack has intellectual and developmental disabilities, which made him vulnerable to provocation by his younger brothers (1 and 2 years his junior). He frequently responded with violence to this provocation, whereupon they would taunt him. This pattern of behavior continued over time, in large part, outside the supervision provided by their mother. Her capacity to supervise them was compromised by the fact that their father had been sent to prison for physically abusing her and Jack. As a result, she needed to work longer hours, thus making matters for her three sons more difficult. Jack was placed in an intensive residential placement where he made very little progress and seemed to spend considerable time developing skills at provoking the front-line staff members into conflict.

Around his eighteenth birthday, the juvenile system felt that he had reached maximum treatment benefit and considered discharging him to an uncertain future. His mother, by now in much better personal circumstances, successfully petitioned the court to become his legal guardian. She then arranged for him to be placed in a group home marked by less structure and supervision. He completed an assessment, which found that his most prioritized PHFs were agency, life, and relatedness. Because he lacked the internal capacity to achieve these PHGs, and because the nature of his placements had meant he focused on very little else, his attempts to achieve one PHG often came into conflict with his attempts to achieve another. He would attempt to exert his agency through yelling at staff and housemates only to then realize that they wanted very little to do with him (signaling problems with relatedness). Every environment he stayed in posed a potential existential threat to his living and surviving. This led to an ongoing pattern of aggression, shame, repentance, attempts to rebuild relationships, etc. Jack had never entirely known a life without violence or the threat of violence. Because of this, trauma-informed GLP implementation had to start slowly, with the staff focusing on safety for self and others within a structured and supervised milieu format. It was ironic that the move from a higher-security setting to a group home in the community had resulted in the very behaviors that had contributed to his initial placement.

As an emerging adult, Jack was still highly dependent on his mother, whose presence had vacillated over the years. Further, the nature of their relationship had changed, through mutual victimization to attempts at reconciliation, to her becoming his guardian. It seemed to Jack that there was a seemingly endless barrage of changes from outside himself, while there were increases in the demands made on him to change. The nature of the many challenges that Jack faced meant that:

- His practical identity changed, in accordance with the environments in which he found himself. For example, he was expected to demonstrate more agency and balance this with the changing role of relatedness in his life. In response, he reexamined his sense of identity and purpose in his life (spirituality).
- His pre-therapy GLP never had vertical or horizontal coherence and was noteworthy for being survival-based.
- He had faced every obstacle a client could possibly experience. He lacked internal and external capacity, had a narrow scope to his GLP, experienced conflicts between his attempts to attain the PHGs most valuable to him, and used inappropriate means to achieve them regularly.

In summary, emerging adults are often:

- More dependent upon their environment and caregivers
- Less established with respect to forming practical identities
- In great need of internal capacities for living independently
- More noticeably influenced by early life trauma and adversity
- Lacking in agency and an internal locus of control

5.8 Case Examples of GLM at a System-Wide Level

Starting Reentry in Prison An attempted escape from a prison caught the attention of the superintendent. In reviewing the case, the superintendent concluded that a greater emphasis on therapy as a means of skill acquisition and rehearsal might have prevented this incident from happening. Very aware that change was needed, she paused intervention services for several weeks and developed a plan for a more seamless transition of clients into the community.

The superintendent took note that the feedback from the incarcerated individuals was that they needed skills for living in the community upon their release, and for practicing effective self-regulation while incarcerated. Thus, she initiated a highly structured skills development program aimed at improving client functioning in these areas, understanding that it would help them to address the PHGs of life, agency, relatedness, inner peace, community, knowledge, mastery at work, and mastery at play. The curricula focused on these areas to address basic skills deficits that everyone (staff and clients) agreed were of primary importance.

As each client neared their release date, they entered an educational group that introduced them to the GLM. Although they did not enter a formal GLM assessment, they engaged in reflective discussion with therapists trained in the GLM, and began to discuss how they could potentially use the GLM during the first days of their reentry into the community and then in more formal treatment once they were released. These discussions were largely informal and helped clients to see how the skills they had developed could be put to use to help them in the future. They also focused on client anxieties and anticipations as they came closer to reentering a community that was ambivalent about having them back.

After their release, the clients were referred to therapists who worked under contract with the correctional system. The therapists would complete a GLM assessment and then work with the clients to develop and implement their GLP. In this way, there could be a smooth transition through a notoriously challenging time in clients' lives.

Ambivalent Return An agency assisted people who returned to the community from prison, drug rehabilitation centers, and similar programs. They developed a guiding document that involved each of the PHGs. Alongside the PHGs were scales from 0 to 10. As part of the initial screening, clients were asked:

- On a scale of 0 to 10, how important is this PHG to you?
- On the same scale of 0 to 10, how confident are you that you can attain it?
- How did you come to choose the numbers that you did?
- With everything that is going on in your life, why did you not score yourself lower on your confidence to make changes in this area?
- What would it take for you to have more confidence in achieving this?

Many will recognize this as a classic approach often described in motivational interviewing texts (Rollnick et al., 2023). The questions are designed to elicit the client's internal motivation to make difficult changes in their life. Similar versions of these scales have been used in a number of GLM workbooks (e.g., Prescott & Dent, 2018; Prescott & Pflugradt, 2024; Yates & Prescott, 2011). From here, the agency would then engage the client in further discussion. Assuming that the client was interested in service, they would then undergo an assessment and enter a broader treatment program.

5.9 Further Reflections on the Challenges of Reentry

Therapists using the GLM often find that it lends itself to a return to the basics of psychotherapy, including positive regard, understanding the processes underlying behaviors, and the importance of simply listening, as the following vignette illustrates.

Eddie grew up in horrific circumstances. He was placed in foster care at age eight and eventually ended up in a high-security juvenile institution where he received little meaningful therapy. He was discharged on his 18th birthday with very little aftercare in place. Within days, he attempted suicide and was placed in a psychiatric hospital. While he was inside, he frequently attempted to barricade himself in his room. When staff would intervene, his sole response was to scream and threaten them with violence. Eddie quickly received a diagnosis of antisocial personality disorder (despite having no convictions as an adult) and was viewed as having no respect or concern for the rights and welfare of others. Having no family, a judge committed him to the care of the state, and he was assigned a legal guardian from a state agency.

Eddie was eventually released into a community-based residential program with specialized staff. Almost as soon as the staff welcomed him to the program, he barricaded himself in his room. Unlike in his previous programs and his hospitalization, the staff instantly understood this behavior as reflective of maladaptive attempts to achieve PHGs such as life and agency. They remained confident that, whatever his diagnosis, he still had some yearning for relatedness. However, he was highly ambivalent about his connections to others, which had virtually always ended in disaster. The staff members took the behaviors very seriously and were always prepared to intervene if safety to Eddie or others became an issue. Just the same, they continued to recognize the underlying search for PHGs that are common to everyone and that they could personally relate to. They also understood that Eddie had experienced very serious earlier life adversity.

Eddie spent his days impressing the staff with his effectiveness at avoiding contact and barricading himself in his room. He could go for long periods of time without eating or using the toilet. During this time, his assigned therapist and members of the staff made periodic offers to talk, engage in collective problem-solving, or any other form of negotiating safely to help Eddie develop a more desirable lifestyle within the program. Importantly, the staff members and therapist abided by the belief that, "If you act like you only have five minutes, it will take all day; but if you act like to have all day it will only take five minutes."

While room barricades in the past had formed a sort of tug-of-war with countless staff, a zero-sum game that no one really won, Eddie's staff in this program simply seemed to drop the metaphorical rope and wait. Eddie became increasingly less interested and came out. Nothing more was said. Eddie's therapist and treatment team simply took the time to talk with him, show him around the program, and get to know him. Eddie's behavior changed dramatically, very quickly. The staff identified things about him that they liked and engaged with him accordingly. He went on to make significant progress in rebuilding his life.

Ironically, when Eddie's therapist asked how it was possible that he had gone from such extreme behaviors to full-fledged treatment engagement, Eddie's only answer was that the staff had simply listened to him, and both understood and respected him in doing so. During those first days, they had not betrayed his evolving trust, and this was enough for him to decide that it was time to become a new person. In the end, it was the simplest therapeutic action that yielded the greatest results: Listening with a goal of understanding.

5.10 Conclusion

The case of Eddie immediately above is emblematic of the challenges that face most clients who attempt to reenter their community. Changes in external circumstances often accompany the need for dramatic internal change. Staying true to the style, spirit, and structure of the GLM practice framework can help clients navigate these turbulent times. Special attention is required to help understand and manage the various barriers that clients often present in the initial stages of therapy. Further case examples illustrating these challenges are presented in Chap. 8.

References

American Psychological Association. (2023). *Inclusive language guide*. (2nd ed.). https://www.apa.org/about/apa/equity-diversity-inclusion/language-guidelines.pdf.

Aos, S., Miller, M., & Drake, E. (2006). Evidence-based public policy options to reduce future prison construction, criminal justice costs, and crime rates (Document No. 06-10-1201). Washington State Institute for Public Policy.

Blasko, B. L., Friedmann, P. D., Rhodes, A. G., & Taxman, F. S. (2015). The parolee–parole officer relationship as a mediator of criminal justice outcomes. *Criminal Justice and Behavior, 42*(7), 722–740. https://doi.org/10.1177/0093854814562642

Crane, J. (2019, July 16). Becoming institutionalized: Incarceration and "slow death." Scientific American. https://items.ssrc.org/insights/becoming-institutionalized-incarceration-and-slow-death/.

Fitch, K. V., Pence, B. W., Rosen, D. L., Miller, V. E., Gaynes, B. N., Swilley-Martinez, M. E., Kavee, A. L., Carey, T. S., Proescholdbell, S. K., & Ranapurwala, S. I. (2024). Suicide mortality among formerly incarcerated people compared with the general population in North Carolina, 2000-2020. *American Journal of Epidemiology, 193*(3), 489–499. https://doi.org/10.1093/aje/kwad214

Harmon, K. (2012, February 4). Brain injury rate seven times higher among U.S. prisoners. Scientific American. https://www.scientificamerican.com/article/traumatic-brain-injury-prison/.

Harris, D. A., & Levenson, J. S. (2020). A framework for post-conviction traumatic stress: Preliminary findings from a focus group of men under community supervision for sex offences. *Psychology, Crime & Law, 28*(3), 241–261. https://doi.org/10.1080/1068316X.2022.2157827

Harris, D. A., Pedneault, A., & Willis, G. (2019). The pursuit of primary human goods in men desisting from sexual offending. *Sexual Abuse, 31*(2), 197–219. https://doi.org/10.1177/1079063217729155. Epub 2017 Sep 5.

Levenson, J. S., Willis, G. M., & Prescott, D. S. (2017). *Trauma-informed care: Transforming treatment for people who have sexually abused*. Safer Society Press.

Maruna, S., LeBel, T. P., Mitchell, N., & Naples, M. (2004). Pygmalion in the reintegration process: Desistance from crime through the looking glass. *Psychology, Crime & Law, 10*(3), 271–281. https://doi.org/10.1080/10683160410001662762

McCartan, K., Prescott, D. S., & Ackerman, A. (2018, September 7). Integration into the community of people who have committed sexual abuse. ATSA Blog. https://blog.atsa.com/2018/09/integration-into-community-of-people.html.

Rollnick, S., Miller, W. R., & Butler, C. C. (2023). *Motivational interviewing in health care: Helping patients change behavior* (2nd ed.). The Guilford Press.

Parhar, K. K., Wormith, J. S., Derkzen, D. M., & Beauregard, A. M. (2008). Offender coercion in treatment: A metaanalysis of effectiveness. *Criminal Justice and Behavior, 35*(9), 1109–1135.

Petrich, D. M., Pratt, T. C., Jonson, C. L., & Cullen, F. T. (2021). Custodial sanctions and reoffending: A meta-analytic review. *Crime and Justice, 50*, 353–424.

Popova, S., Lange, S., Bekmuradov, D., Mihic, A., & Rehm, J. (2011). Fetal alcohol spectrum disorder prevalence estimates in correctional systems: A systematic literature review. *Canadian Journal of Public Health, 102*(5), 336–340. https://doi.org/10.1007/BF03404172

Prescott, D. S., & Dent, T. M. (2018). *Becoming who I want to be: A good lives model workbook for young women*. Safer Society Press.

Prescott, D. S., & Pflugradt, D. M. (2024). *Becoming the man I want to be* (2nd ed.). Safer Society Press.

Purvis, M., Ward, T., & Shaw, S. (2013). *Applying the good lives model to the case management of sexual offenders*. Safer Society Press.

Ryan, R. M., & Deci, E. L. (2000). Self-determination theory and the facilitation of intrinsic motivation, social development, and well-being. *American Psychologist, 55*(1), 68–78. https://doi.org/10.1037/0003-066X.55.1.68

Ryan, R. M., & Deci, E. L. (2017). *Self-determination theory: Basic psychological needs in motivation, development, and wellness*. Guilford Press.

Sheldon, K. M. (2020). Going the distance on the Pacific Crest Trail: The vital role of identified motivation. *Motivation Science, 6*(2), 177–181. https://doi.org/10.1037/mot0000147

Smith, P., Goggin, C., & Gendreau, P. (2002). *The effects of prison sentences and intermediate sanctions on recidivism: General effects and individual differences*. Solicitor General Canada.

Ward, T., Willis, G. M., & Prescott, D. S. (2024). The rehabilitation of corrections clients: Good lives and risk reduction. In G. M. Davies & A. R. Beech (Eds.), *Forensic psychology: Crime, justice, law, interventions* (pp. 511–531). Wiley.

Willis, G. M. (2018). Why call someone by what we don't want them to be? The ethics of labeling in forensic/correctional psychology. *Psychology, Crime & Law, 24*(7), 727–743. https://doi.org/10.1080/1068316X.2017.1421640

Wilson, R. J., Cortoni, F., & McWhinnie, A. J. (2009). Circles of support & accountability: A Canadian national replication of outcome findings. *Sexual Abuse: Journal of Research and Treatment, 21*(4), 412–430. https://doi.org/10.1177/1079063209347724

Yates, P. M., & Prescott, D. S. (2011). *Building a better life: A good lives and self-regulation workbook*. Safer Society Press.

Chapter 6
Community Interventions

6.1 Introduction

How should we act when people who committed crimes, such as sex offenses, return to society? What is the potential of community interventions based on the good lives model (GLM)? In this chapter, the application of the GLM in structuring supervision for individuals on parole or probation is explored, along with implications for community engagement. The ways in which the GLM can facilitate effective and individually engaging community interventions are emphasized.

An illustration will specifically focus on a Belgian case example in which a risk perspective is embedded in a human rights and social work perspective. Tenets of the strengths-based practice (SBP) (Simmons et al., 2016) are used to inform three dynamic stages of implementing the GLM in community interventions: assessment, the development of a good lives plan (GLP), and therapy (Ward et al., 2007). The chapter also considers good practices and provides examples of implementation that may inspire therapists working with the GLM.

6.2 Forensic Outpatient Services: In Society, on Parole, or Probation

The landscape of structuring supervision for individuals on parole or probation is very diverse. Worldwide, it has been organized both in- and outside of the justice system, depending on historical choices (Giulini et al., 2020). This chapter will look at a contemporary example in the context of continental Europe, specifically Flanders, the northern region of Belgium.

T. Ward et al., *The Good Lives Model of Correctional Rehabilitation*, Advances in Preventing and Treating Violence and Aggression,
https://doi.org/10.1007/978-3-031-95559-4_6

In Flanders, forensic social work and mental health care for people who have committed sexual crimes and are on parole or probation is organized outside the justice system. Both in psychiatric hospitals and in community teams (outpatient services), cooperation agreements between the national government and local communities serve to develop a specialized care network for the guidance and treatment of people who commit sex offenses (Verellen & De Boeck, 2020). Most people who are convicted reside in society on parole or on probation and have therapy in the facilities mentioned above.

This practice differs from the work of probation officers. Because the centers for specialized therapy are subsidized by the ministry of welfare and health, it is part of the social work and health care field of practice. The rules on client confidentiality are stricter as compared to those followed by probation officers. There is no duty to report criminal acts or a failure to comply with the conditions, although there are obligations to assure care for victims and to break confidentiality when people are in danger (Versweyvelt et al., 2018).

6.3 Risk Perspective Embedded in a Human Right and Social Work Perspective

Forensic work in Flanders focuses beyond a risk perspective and combines welfare rights with relapse prevention (Wanzeele & Oltenfreiter, 2020, Ward & Brown, 2004). From 2000 onward, forensic social work in Flanders has been defined as a welfare-oriented approach in relation to criminal justice interventions (Bouverne-De Bie, 2002; Naessens, 2023). Welfare goals related to human rights and human dignity have a central place in this approach (Meyvis et al., 2012; Van Garsse, 2012).

Human rights and human dignity, when put into practice and structurally embedded, are key elements of a social work perspective (Borowski, 2022; Garrett, 2024; Naessens, 2023; see Chap. 1). From this perspective, criminal behavior is considered as a complex interplay of individual, social, environmental, and systemic factors (Taylor & Frost, 2017). Because it is based on a compassionate, rehabilitative, and preventative point of view, practice takes a holistic, person-centered approach to understanding and addressing criminal behavior. It focuses on understanding the causes of criminal behavior, supporting individuals in their rehabilitation, and advocating for systemic changes that reduce inequality and improve social conditions (Fenton, 2013; Naessens, 2023; Taylor & Frost, 2017).

The GLM is also based on human rights and dignity perspectives (see Chap. 1; Ward, 2009, 2011). In that sense, it aligns well with practices of forensic social work and mental health care. A move toward reducing discrimination, working collaboratively, taking a desistance approach, and promoting good lives gradually became the new standard of forensic therapy (Ward, 2011). Based on this shift, traditional (risk-oriented) approaches in the forensic field were increasingly questioned and criticized. An example is the "offense chain" model that has long been considered the standard way of applying cognitive behavioral therapy (Marshall et al., 1999). The focus on risk leads to avoidance goals that are not connected to individuals' prioritized primary goods (Mann et al., 2004, Ward et al., 2006). Therapy using an offense chain model approach requires individuals to memorize and present this chain to therapists, focusing primarily on identifying ways to avoid risk factors. When questioned about risk factors such as associating with antisocial peers, the reasons why they were motivated to spend time with such "bad friends" were typically overlooked. This often led to a gap between "what they should tell" and "what they like to tell."

Based on human rights and human dignity, the GLM was increasingly offered as a way to complement the "what works" and "who works" principles (Willis & Ward, 2024). In this way, the focus on relapse prevention became inseparable from addressing well-being related concerns and discovering strengths by means of approach goals (Ward et al., 2007; Wanzeele & Oltenfreiter, 2020). In conclusion, a social work and strengths-based approach aligns well with the theoretical and practical framework of the GLM.

6.4 Using the Strength-Based Practice (SBP) to Implement the GLM

The SBP framework (Simmons et al., 2016, 2021) focuses on promoting individual well-being by changing behavior, reducing social problems and enforcing social change. Core values and constructs are resilience, hope, empowerment, self-determination, client involvement, and looking at the person-in-environment (Franklin, 2015; Simmons et al., 2016, 2021). SBP shares a strong conceptual alignment with the GLM, with both models focusing on the positive aspects of individuals' lives rather than solely on deficits or problems. The SBP and GLM emphasize that people are primarily motivated by personal values and the pursuit of meaningful, fulfilling lives. Both approaches concentrate on building individual capacities, rather than correcting deficits, and on positive development and resilience in order to achieve adaptive changes in individuals' behavior. As SBP and GLM both underline the ethical and therapeutic value of personal autonomy, both argue that individuals should be active agents in their processes of change.

Manthey et al. (2011: 135) distilled the strengths principles of Saleebey (2006) and Rapp et al. (2005) into eight crucial tenets of SBP (Simmons et al., 2021). These were developed as a response to the observation that many programs that claimed to be strengths-based were still primarily problem focused (Douglas et al., 2014; Rapp & Goscha, 2006; Simmons et al., 2021). These principles are useful to check the strengths-based level of a program. The eight tenets are:

1. *Goal-oriented*: attention on what people want to achieve in life and keeping the focus on reaching positive goals. Goals are associated with secondary goods and good lives plans (see Chap. 1).

2. *Needs-oriented* (or goods-oriented): a continuous focus on primary goods, their associated secondary goods, and the development of a plan to achieve them.
3. *Strengths-oriented*: strengths are defined in this context as the personal and social capital required to reach a person's goals.
4. *Context-oriented*: strengths relate to individual characteristics, important others, and the environment of communities and society. This context should be involved in all stages of implementation.
5. *Hope-oriented*: inducing hope through all stages of the change process (Snyder et al., 2018).
6. *Therapeutic relationship*: during all stages of implementation, the therapist has to

   "reflect authentic warmth; listen well; affirm the client's perspective, hopes, and capacities to overcome any difficulties; and, whenever possible, share and generate power with their client" (Simmons et al., From Theory to Practice section, para. 4, 2021).

7. *Trauma-sensitive*: trauma symptoms can become barriers to building good lives and therefore are treated in order to promote adaptive coping, creating conditions that reduce risk for recidivism (Harris & Levenson, 2020; Levenson et al., 2017).
8. *Future-oriented*: It is always possible to discover more strengths (Manthey et al., 2011). The stages of the implementation of the GLM are not linear, but implemented in a dynamic way, because new information in every step could contribute to building a (future) life adapted to the most important goods.

The rest of this chapter highlights how these eight tenets of SBP (Simmons et al., 2021) can guide the implementation of the GLM in forensic outpatient services.

6.5 Stages of Implementation of the GLM in the Community

The course of GLM-directed community interventions occurs in three dynamic stages (Ward, Mann, & Gannon, 2007): assessment, the development of a GLP, and therapy. Throughout these stages, the following practical examples highlight good practice when implementing the GLM.

Throughout the stages, it is important to follow the tenets of SBP, with attention to orientation to goals, needs, strengths, hope, context, therapeutic relationship, trauma, and future orientation. This structure will be used in the following description of each of the three stages of GLM implementation.

6.5.1 Assessment

Assessment is an exploration stage using a GLM interview (Barnao, 2013; Purvis et al., 2011; Yates et al., 2010). The goal is to gain insight into the perceived importance of the primary goods, how they are met (secondary goods), and which goods played a central role in criminal behavior. This interview must start from a genuine interest in the person, rather than giving priority to the criminal acts. What does this person want in life? What goods are most important? What stands in the way of securing these goods? How has the person been able to fulfill this particular good in the past? What strengths has that person used?

In a multidisciplinary team meeting, professionals analyze the information gathered in the GLM mapping table (Appendix c; see Chap. 3) and discuss their interpretation of the primary goods that are currently most important to the individual and those that were connected with the crime(s). This leads to a collectively shared hypothesis of the most important primary goods for the individual. The therapist asks for feedback from the client in order to reach a jointly supported analysis.

The GLM mapping table and the supported analysis are used to inform a case formulation (Yates et al., 2010). In this process, the offense(s) (and other secondary goods, including risk factors) are surveyed within the client's life and context. Developing an understanding of an individual's prioritized primary goods and their associated secondary goods, along with their obstacles and strengths serves to clarify the mechanisms of their offending.

The SBP principles can be useful to formulate questions for the GLM assessment:

- Are the client's life goals clear? Are these a translation of the primary goods?
- Is there an understanding of the relationship between the client's primary and secondary goods, including those connected to the crime(s)?
- Are the strengths of the client identified and connected with the primary goods?
- Have the client's significant others been involved in the assessment?
- Has the client's hope for change been assessed and linked to their primary goods and strengths?
- Have the first steps for a strong therapeutic alliance been taken during the assessment?
- Is there a focus on trauma and its importance as an obstacle related to offending?
- Has the outcome of the assessment been discussed with the client?

Assessment is strongly influenced by the type of questions that are asked. In a strength-based approach the questions create space for clients to disclose their goals in life. Exemplary questions include the following (quoted from the GLM tool kit developed by Barnao (2013; see Chap. 3):

When you were young, what did you dream about becoming later in life? What were the goals that you had for yourself? What did you do to meet those goals? Were some goals more important to you than others? Which ones were and why? What got in the way of meeting your goals?

If you could be anyone at all (e.g., people you know, famous or infamous people, fictional characters) who would you most want to be like? Why? Who would you least want to be like? Why?

What sort of life would you like for yourself in the future? What would you like to achieve? What have you always wanted to achieve?

If you could wake up 1 day and things were just as you wanted them to be what would it be like? Where would you be? What would you be doing? How would you be feeling? Who would you be with? What things wouldn't you be doing?

These questions focus on positive goals that the client wants to reach. These aspirations (i.e., secondary goods) are explored with a view to understanding which primary good(s) the person was trying to fulfill through this goal. For example, when a 19-year-old person has the goal of becoming a professional soccer player, what primary good(s) is being sought? Does he want to be an expert in play? Does he want more agency by earning money? Does he want to be part of a group (a team)? The assessment should provide this information, which is discussed with the client, to reach a jointly supported understanding. Thus, the goals of the client, formulated in terms of secondary goods, are linked to the corresponding primary goods that explain the needs connected with these goals. During the GLM mapping table and/or in the case formulation is the time to provide and discuss an overview of the PHGs (and their importance), the secondary goods, the strengths, the obstacles, and the link between them and with the crime(s).

A central focus during assessment is detecting these *needs* or prioritized primary goods that will later help inform the development of the person's GLP. Questions should elicit information about these primary goods. Useful questions include (quoted from the GLM tool kit developed by Barnao (2013):

> Tell me a bit about yourself and your life just before you came into hospital/service. (e.g., What were you doing? What did you enjoy doing? Who did you spend your time with? What was important to you?)

There are many methods to carry out such an assessment. One example is good lives music (Wanzeele & Severs, 2020), a novel approach to GLM assessment which is described in Box 6.1.

Box 6.1

Good lives music is a useful method for group therapy for persons in detention. Because music is universal and a way of connecting people, it has proven to be a useful means for people to express themselves in a non-threatening way (Mehr et al., 2019). During the sessions, therapists ask participants to choose songs that are important to them, that are related to memories, that correspond with their dreams about the future, etc. Participants listen together to the songs that were chosen after which a group discussion takes place.

Talking about music provides an opportunity to explore the goods that are most important to the person. This is illustrated by the following two examples, obtained from clients in the Brussels prison (Wanzeele & Severs, 2020):

> When I hear this song ("Undertaker" by Aimée Allen) it reminds me of my mother cookin' and singin' in the kitchen. For me it is important to know what I used to like, not only what went wrong in the past. This coziness and warmth at home I really liked a lot. (Wanzeele & Severs, 2020: 6)

The prioritized PHG was identified as relatedness, more specifically with his mother. The participant talked about the importance of loving your most valuable family members. His comments also pointed to a feeling of pleasure derived from being in a warm and comfortable situation.

> I want you to discover this song and its lyrics (Linval Thompson ft. Bounty Killer & Sizzla, "Train to Zion"). It's all about peace, love and revolution. This is also the message I want to send out. (Wanzeele & Severs, 2020: 7)

This person wanted to fulfill a purpose in life: spreading this message to others to create a better world, reflecting spirituality as a primary good.

A key objective of GLM assessment is to gain understanding of the primary goods that the person was trying to fulfill directly or indirectly through their criminal behavior. According to the GLM, a person's offending is an attempt to satisfy legitimate primary goods, but they are going about it in the wrong way. Through conversation and/or the use of more creative methods, the connection between criminal activities and the pursuit of primary goods is clarified. Identifying which PHG a person experiences as most important in life contributes to a successful assessment, because these are considered priorities when developing a GLP. A primary good that is related to several secondary goods makes this good more important to focus on.

Client *strengths* are often overlooked due to a tendency for clinicians working within the criminal justice domain to focus primarily on risk factors (Mann et al., 2004). A growing focus on strengths has led to the development of specific tools that are used to map strengths in an individual's life (see Chap. 3). Strengths may be protective factors for relapse prevention. For example, self-control (internal strength) and a prosocial network (external strength) are both protective factors against reoffending in violent risk areas (de Vogel et al., 2012). Strengths include more than just protective factors, e.g., being good at playing music is a strength but not a protective factor. When working with people who committed violent crimes, the structured assessment of protective factors for violence risk (SAPROF) categorizes these factors well (de Vogel et al., 2012). Protective factors can be seen as domains within which there are multiple strengths, e.g., as empathy contains cognitive, emotional, and compassionate empathy, one person may have strong cognitive empathy, but could develop a better emotional and compassionate empathy. Discussing strengths with clients can increase their motivation for engaging in therapy. An orientation to strengths during the assessment phase means that current strengths can be deployed in the construction of the person's GLP, with links made to the person's prioritized primary goods.

To detect external strengths, it is important to involve individuals who can play prosocial roles in the person's life. Often, the assessment is seen as a task of therapists, at best in consultation with the client involved. But why not let the important others—the context of this client—contribute to the assessment of strengths and all other aspects of a GLM assessment? A context may include family, friends, or other caregivers. There are different methods to gain perspective into the network of the client, including ecological maps. Family treatment or family group conferences (Edwards & Parkinson, 2018) are methods that fit when involving more than one's family.

Having identified some important considerations in carrying out a GLM assessment drawing on the tenets of SBP, it is time to consider how a multidisciplinary team might undertake this process. The following four steps may be useful:

1. After going through the initial interviews, team members (with different professional backgrounds) carry out a joint assessment. The first step in this multidisciplinary assessment is collectively filling out the GLM mapping table (see Chap. 3). The diverse views of different staff members have great value: e.g., what is similar or complementary in terms of information provided by the support worker or the creative therapist? What differences are there in the information that has been gathered?
2. The second step is a joint discussion integrating the information obtained from the mapping table process. This integration is grounded in a dynamic interaction between the different team members who are trained in the GLM and its implementation. This training is crucial for developing high-quality assessments (Prescott et al., 2022). The main primary goods, the connection to criminal behavior, the connected obstacles (see Chaps. 1 and 2) and strengths are concisely summarized in a GLM mapping table.
3. Next, this (preliminary) synthesis is summarized by the team members in a case formulation, in which the connections between the PHGs, secondary goods, and offending behavior and contexts are formulated in a narrative form that is accessible for the client.
4. Finally, the assessment is shared with the client to test whether it is consistent with the client's perception. The GLM mapping table and the case formulation are adjusted and fine-tuned by the team and client, if necessary.

It should go without saying that the client should be an active participant at the helm. In this way, it is important to avoid talking over anyone's head, and to engage in dialogue with the client. All conversations with other people (e.g., family, friends, etc.) about the client only happen with the permission of the person. By doing so, we aim to maximize agency and reduce paternalism. How can important others contribute? Those who know the client well could participate in the assessment. They could also be involved in discussions about the case formulation or how they might support the client in the plan for change (GLP).

Involving important others in this process may contribute to hope for change. The adult hope scale (AHS) measures hope as a motivational state based on a sense of successful goal-directed energy and planning to meet goals (Snyder et al., 1991, 2018). The goal-directed energy is related to the primary good of agency. The scale measures whether the client is able to pursue their goals energetically, has been successful in life, has met the goals that were set, and was prepared for the future by past experiences. In the planning, items focus on the ability to think of pathways to get out of trouble or to obtain the things in life that are important for the client.

Based on the assessment through the mapping table and/or the case formulation, it can be useful to consider which domains people will trust in a positive future. These domains can be labeled with "H" in the mapping table. Assessing hope in this way provides information about the person's motivation and may be useful in intervention planning. Hope for change in obtaining a certain good can be seen as a strength that a person can draw on when working on their GLP.

Giving attention to hope during the assessment can contribute to a *therapeutic relationship* that induces hope (Saleebey, 2006). The quality of the therapeutic relationship, along with the environment in which therapy takes place, play an important role in the creation of a safe environment in which the client is supported and empowered (Simmons et al., 2021). People who are on probation should experience the engagement of those who provide therapy from the very outset.

Three elements are important to focus on:

1. Meeting environments: The building, the accessibility, and the therapy room are all elements of the environment that influence the degree to which a person feels comfortable. A therapy room should be designed in such a way that people feel comfortable and safe (Haight et al., 2002; Simmons et al., 2021).
2. Attitude: From the start of therapy, clients should be welcomed by the therapist and treated with empathy, warmth, and respect (Marshall et al., 2011).
3. Content: A basic element of implementation of the GLM is the content of what we talk about with our clients. Focusing on what is really important to them helps to strengthen the therapeutic alliance (Barnao et al., 2015; Ross et al., 2008).

The client should notice some crucial things:

- My therapist is paying attention to what I really care about.
- My therapist is willing to help me find a way forward without judging me while remaining clear about the unacceptability of the criminal acts.
- After all these questions my therapist gives me something back that I recognize or that can be modified if I don't identify with it.
- My therapist will not make decisions over my head.

It is important for the therapist to show an understanding of the client's suffering. Recently, there has been an increased focus on the importance of trauma, because many of those who have committed crimes have experienced trauma (Cantürk et al., 2021, Levenson et al., 2016). The impacts of trauma can pose obstacles to the attainment of one or more PHGs such as relatedness, inner peace, or happiness. Trauma should be considered in understanding risk and protective factors, highlighted by a recent study showed that suggests people convicted for sexual offenses indicated that

> exploring and processing past trauma would aid them in developing new coping skills to avoid recidivism (Grady et al., 2022:16).

For example, in the case of substance use being used to satisfy the primary good of inner peace that has been undermined due to trauma, a plan to address the substance abuse needs to be built into the person's GLP.

Grady et al. (2022:20) indicate that

> A movement toward more trauma-informed SOTX [sex-offending specific treatment programming] contextualizes offending as a symptomatic constellation of underlying problems, rather than simply a behavior to be extinguished. Obviously, prevention of future sex crimes is the most salient goal of treatment, and this objective might be more successfully achieved by using more trauma-informed RNR interventions.

The analysis of risk factors, and the link with trauma and the related PHGs, could support this type of intervention. Trauma-informed sex offending treatment has been developed to recognize trauma symptoms as it addresses factors signaled by dynamic risk factors (Levenson et al., 2017). These risk factors are obstacles to the fulfillment of primary goods and, as such, are important to understand.

Prescott and Levenson (in press), have formulated some important questions that therapists should consider when thinking about the role of trauma and adverse events in the client's life and their relationship to risk (see Chap. 2):

What is the story, or narrative, of this risk factor in the client's life?
How have adverse events, including cultural adversity and prior experiences with the legal system, contributed to the role of this risk factor in the client's life?
How has the client come to view the world? What kinds of cognitive schemas do the client have about the world? How have these schemas contributed to risk?
What kinds of cognitive schemas has the client developed about themselves? As someone who is broken? Who has to fight back against others? Who has to take what he wants in an unkind world? How have these schemas contributed to risk?
How does the client understand the role of this risk factor in their life?
To what extent are they able to observe and work with this risk factor?
In what ways has this risk factor represented an obstacle to living a better life? (Prescott and Levenson, in press, Conclusion section, para.1)

It is important to detect and determine obstacles and replace them with other, more appropriate, means (Purvis et al., 2011). By explicitly indicating trauma in the GLM mapping table (see Appendix 3 and Chap. 3), e.g., using the reference "T," its impact can be better understood. When the impacts of trauma are recognized as obstacles, it highlights the role that trauma plays in a person's ability to satisfy primary goods, especially in their offending.

During this assessment the goal is to engage people for therapy, in which trauma-informed care could play a role. Responsivity is

> consistent with a trauma-informed approach, which focuses on establishing a safe therapeutic alliance so that clients can develop the trust needed to begin the challenging and often painful work of self-exploration, personal growth, cognitive change, and internal regulation capacity (Grady et al., 2022:17).

In addition to looking at the past, looking ahead requires an increasing focus throughout the conversations. This also means taking time to explore. The alliance between therapist and client must be given time to develop. Primary goods are not always immediately apparent, and the therapist needs a certain willingness to discover them, trusting in the flow of the process.

One should never take the interpretation of the information as fixed. It remains dynamic and can be adjusted or refuted during each stage based on new insights or new information. This open-minded attitude is necessary to maximize the client's agency in this process. Therefore, it is crucial to check the interpretation of the information gathered during the assessment with the client. In this sense, case formulation can be thought of as a set of hypotheses that are checked with the person in order to have the strongest possible impact on the future.

6.5.2 Good Lives Plan (GLP)

A GLP is based on the assessment (Yates et al., 2010; see also Chaps. 1 and 2). It can be assumed that the person's previous life plan was problematic in certain ways, often containing elements that contributed to problems and criminal behavior. At the core of this stage, clinicians should work in close cooperation with the client to explore socially appropriate and adaptive pathways to primary goods. Primary goods are linked to specific goals in the short, medium, and long terms. Each step in the GLP constitutes a building block for the next step. The final goal is for the person to achieve their version of a fulfilling life that doesn't involve further offending.

A central question at this stage is whether the construction of the GLP is SPB-oriented. One way of aligning the development of a GLP with the SPB principles is to consider the following supplementary questions:

- Are the goals in the GLP formulated in a specific, measurable, achievable, relevant, time-bound (SMART) way?
- Does the plan start with attending to the (most important) primary good(s)?
- Are detected strengths linked to the goals, and do the goals include developing new strengths?
- Are the external strengths in the person's life included in the plan?
- Does the client experience hope for achieving the goals in the plan?
- Is the client the owner of the plan?
- Is treatment of trauma included in the plan when it is assessed to be a (repeated) obstacle?
- Does drafting the plan give new insights that change the plan?

In order to formulate goals that fit with the client's needs, the goals should be formulated in a SMART way (Doran, 1981; Locke & Latham, 2002). Using SMART features in setting goals can enhance motivation (Bandura, 1986), making it more likely that the person will achieve their goals. Some more specific guidelines on how to develop SMART GLM goals are provided below:

- *Specific*: Be detailed on what to accomplish and on who should be involved. Be clear about the time frame and the location. Be attentive to conditions that should be fulfilled in order to reach the goal. Focus on the reason why this goal is pursued, and link with the primary goods.

- *Measurable*: Define the starting point and the point of achieving the goal. Identify what is needed to reach the goal and how you will know if the goal has been achieved.
- *Attainable*: Discuss whether the goal is acceptable and achievable for the client. Are there some other aspects of achievable you might want to consider? For example, any constraints in the person's living environment or difficulties with internal capacity?
- *Relevant*: Be sure the goal is fulfilling the primary goods that are intended.
- *Time-bound*: Define a period of time in which the goal could be achieved. A timeline should be realistic and flexible. Make priorities about which secondary goods should be addressed first.

A GLP revolves around the person's most heavily weighted primary goods (linking to their practical identity), and it encompasses a search for alternative ways to fulfill these in a prosocial way. Designing concrete steps to acquire new skills and abilities is, therefore, centered on the person's goals and the fulfillment of their most important primary goods. Gradually this can extend to reaching other primary goods.

Through therapy, people who have offended should gain

> awareness and understanding of what goods and problems were associated with his offending, and therefore what capabilities treatment supplied [them] with to resolve these problems (Ward et al., 2007:104).

The connection to criminal behavior is essential: looking for alternatives (secondary goods) to fulfill the primary good that was directly or indirectly related to offending and equipping the person with the internal and external capabilities to achieve their goals, is linked to addressing dynamic risk factors (see Chap. 2). For example, when a young adult male joins a gang to fulfill the need for community, a prosocial fulfillment of that need, e.g., by getting involved in the local soccer team, could be an alternative to distance himself from the gang. This is only possible if the individual can fulfill the underlying primary good(s) for that secondary good. This positively oriented approach helps to reduce risk.

Achieving goals that are oriented to the most important primary goods in the plan requires conscious attention to the strengths that characterize the client. For example, if a person involved in organized crime is able to plan, divide, and manage tasks very well, these skills may serve equally well in working toward a steady, prosocial job. A strengths-based approach involves aiming to use the plan to reinforce existing strengths and develop new ones. For example, someone with limited social skills and a desire for relatedness and being part of a community can include social skills training and participation in social activities as a step in the plan.

When looking for suitable activities, further areas of interest may appear and reflect client strengths. For example, someone may be interested in a cooking class because they already feel confident in their abilities in this area. Discovering what the person is already capable of or what strengths lie in the person or in the environment is continued in the further development of the GLM. A context that is supportive is a protective factor (de Vries Robbé et al., 2015). It is worth exploring with the client whether they want to involve a team to help think about and co-create the plan. Examples of this are found in therapy for youth and adolescents who commit sex offenses, e.g., family group conferences in South Africa (Gxubane, 2016) apply a restorative justice perspective that connects clients in treatment with people they have harmed to come to decisions about recovery together. In the Netherlands, at "de Horizon" (Munninghoff, 2021), a good lives team is assembled around the young person to help implement some of the goals. A similar good lives team approach can be found in the G-Map-approach in the UK, an implementation of the GLM with youth who sexually offended (Fortune et al., 2014).

Therapist and client should work together to identify past choices related to criminal behavior and how they may be connected to the client's most important primary goods (Purvis et al., 2011). In addition, it important to recognize the aspects for which the client experiences the greatest hope for positive change. For example, if agency is the good that the client was trying to fulfill through their criminal behavior and the analysis shows that they feel hope for change in finding a job that really fits, then the job search can be included as one of the first steps in the plan to strive for a sense of agency.

The therapeutic relationship is ultimately tested in the preparation and development of the GLP. Can the client put enough trust in the therapist to receive support in constructing the plan? People have the right to decide on what is really important for them, which is crucial to harnessing intrinsic motivation (Yates, 2009). The central question becomes whether the client actually owns the plan?

Developing a GLP with people in detention has shown that a plan motivates people to follow therapy (Fox & Freestone, 2008). The good lives and development (GLAD) scheme has been used as a supporting service to the treatment framework inside prison, with targets being collaboratively identified between the person in prison and a team of penitentiary officers and psychological staff (Wood, 2015). One of the conclusions based on an evaluation of this scheme was that the potential progress lies in ensuring that a GLP is set collaboratively (Fox & Freestone, 2008). The level of collaboration that the client experiences should always be checked to maximize the person's engagement.

When trauma caused by childhood adversity is detected during the assessment phase, its impact should be considered in the planning stage, i.e., in the formulation of the GLP. Childhood adversity, as an obstacle to attaining primary goods, is associated with mental health problems and adult criminality (Harlow, 1999; Messina et al., 2007). Trauma-informed care (TIC)

> can be integrated into common programme models or theories of practice, including relapse prevention, cognitive behavioral therapy, the Good Lives Model and Risk-Need-Responsivity models. TIC simply delivers clinical services in a way that recognises the prevalence and impact of early trauma on behavior across the lifespan (Levenson, 2014:18).

Thus, principles of TIC should be integrated within the GLM framework, including in the formulation of the GLP. For example, the plan may contain a response to attachment-based strategies and linked to any trauma that may be detected. Ainsworth et al. (1978) identified three major attachment patterns, referred to as balanced (B), distancing (A), and preoccupied (C). Baim and Morrison (2011) developed an attachment-based practice to promote positive change by challenging the pattern that is detected. When an A or C strategy is identified, the plan focuses on a more balanced strategy. With the A strategy, a person exhibits avoidance behavior, making connection with the trauma difficult. With the C strategy, a person is overwhelmed and preoccupied by the trauma. Both strategies can lead to challenging behavior and are obstacles in dealing with the trauma and in satisfying primary goods such as inner peace. The ideal parent figure (IPF) method, eye movement desensitization and reprocessing (EMDR), attachment-based family therapy (ABFT) or psychodrama are some of the methods that can be used to reshape either strategy into a B strategy where processing of the trauma takes place and the person can move forward with the relevant knowledge and experience from this trauma (Baim et al., 2002).

In this stage, intervention planning inevitably carries an orientation toward the future. To realize behavioral change in the future, the plan should be supported by both therapist and client, with at least some expectation and hope for change on both sides.

6.5.3 Therapy

When a GLP has been completed with the client, the first activities can be scheduled. During this stage, activities accumulate and are put to the test during and outside of therapy sessions. Each activity should be accompanied by an evaluation, discussed by the therapist and the client. Do the activities contribute to a better life for the person? Do they contribute to relapse prevention?

In this stage, we examine how putting the GLP into practice through therapy aligns with the SBP principles mentioned above. The following questions can serve as a guide:

- Does the client reach the goals that were put forward?
- Do the actions contribute to fulfilling the (most import) primary goods in a pro-social way?
- Are strengths used to reach the goals?
- Are external strengths in the person's life included in realizing the plan?
- Does the client experience more hope for a positive future after fulfilling goods through realizing steps of the GLP?
- What does the client gain from experiencing a warm therapeutic relationship?
- Is coping with trauma possible?
- Are new strengths discovered through this stage?

In this final stage, the goals from the plan should be evaluated: Were they achieved? To what extent? Were there any obstacles that stood in the way? If necessary, new goals may be formulated. This would mean going back to the planning stage. The plan is the basis for this evaluation. In the GLP template (see Chap. 3) it is useful to provide space where the evaluation can be described. The question of whether the goal was achieved cannot always be answered with a simple yes or no. A qualitative assessment of this question may also lead to new steps or revising the plan. If everything seems to be on track for goal attainment, a comprehensive evaluation is not necessary after every step. Still, an ongoing evaluation is appropriate to make timely adjustments.

The GLP template (see Chap. 3) or the case formulation can be used to evaluate whether the needs of the person, i.e., the primary goods, are now being fulfilled in a prosocial way. The most central goal of the GLM is apositive, prosocial fulfillment of the primary goods, especially those that played a role in offending. A GLP is not successful until this fulfillment becomes a reality. The ways in which the primary goods were fulfilled are evaluated, and the newly gained secondary goods that contribute to this in a prosocial way are considered successful. As argued in Chap. 2, DRF play useful role in signaling what PHGs are the focus of a person's offending-related behavior and their life at the time of their offending.

This is the time to evaluate the strengths that were deployed and the obstacles that were tackled. The latter should be evaluated by carrying out a risk assessment of dynamic risk factors. For example, a measure such as the STABLE 2007 (Fernandez et al., 2014), a dynamic measure of risk factors for sexual offending used with adult males, would be appropriate to assess risk in individuals who have committed sexual offenses.

Evaluations should also check whether the internal and external strengths already available to the person were used. Did these strengths contribute to achieving the goal or was more needed to achieve this goal? For example, it could be that someone labeled with autism spectrum disorder (ASD) has used their cognitive skills (internal strength) to learn new social skills through social skills training, but the person failed to participate in social activities. This should be further investigated in that case. It may be that the client was burdened by overstimulation, making social activities not feasible. The plan can be adjusted accordingly to tackle this obstacle.

A strengths-based approach supports maximizing prosocial influences in a person's life. A supportive context is a protective factor (de Vries Robbé et al., 2015). More than co-developing the GLP, an individual's supports can be part of the implementation process, acting as an external strength to realize the plan. For example, a man who was imprisoned multiple times for violent crimes and theft that resulted in estrangement from most of his family might be in contact with his brother who is not involved in offending behavior. The brother indicates he is available to provide practical support upon release, but the client is late for an appointment due to traffic problems. He did not notify his brother, leading to the brother telling him not to visit anymore. The trust has been broken, which signifies a change in the availability of the trustworthy other. Restoration in the relationship is needed to maintain the external strength.

Plan implementation is not carried out in isolation from the immediate environment, neither is it done in isolation from the broader environment, i.e., society. Thus, societal factors can have a tangible impact. Think, for instance, about the impact of war on the individual and their basic needs. Another example might be the closure of a factory that leaves thousands of workers on the street. The opposite is also true: a society that develops facilities and networks that help prevent social problems can also have a structural impact on the primary goods of the life of many. This transcends the individual but when structural obstacles recur, it also makes sense for clinicians to take them on through signaling, public education, and social action where possible (Murray & Hick, 2012).

Given that having hope, maintaining hope, and growing hope during therapy produces more positive outcomes of therapy (Burlingame & Jensen, 2017; Snyder et al., 2018), it is important to follow up on this. One way to measure if there is positive change in hope, is implementing the AHS in a continuous way (Snyder et al., 1991, 2018). The scale can be used at different times in therapy to check in which areas the person's hope is evolving.

It follows that as primary goods become fulfilled, the person experiences a better life, is less likely to engage in antisocial or maladaptive behavior, and has greater confidence in a positive future. For the therapist, it is useful to see which steps in the plan have the most effect on hope. Based on monitoring hope, this can be checked and discussed with the client.

When the client experiences an increase in their well-being from working through their GLP, they may experience even greater trust in the therapist and service involved. The therapeutic relationship is then strengthened. Even if this occurs in the context of mandated care/support, a client may experience the benefit to their own life. This experience can help them learn to trust others. It can enable people to seek help more quickly if they get into trouble again. Entering a therapeutic relationship that incorporates attention to well-being can thus become an anchor to strengthen the quality of other relationships. In this way, the client learns to engage in other relationships even during therapy, with the prospect of continuing this in a qualitative manner with important others in their life.

Implementation of the plan may include coping with trauma. After putting a trauma-informed GLP into practice (Levenson, 2014), the extent to which the obstacles associated with trauma still stand in the way of satisfying certain primary goods can be evaluated and taken into account. Their attachment strategies (Baim & Morrison, 2011) can also be examined. Does the client, after treatment, succeed in adopting a more balanced (B) strategy? If so, how does this contribute to a higher level of well-being, i.e., access to the primary goods?

Putting a plan into practice means the future is now. When planned steps of the GLP are successful, people often discover that they have much more human capital than they anticipated. For example, a person may join a sports club to satisfy the good of being part of a community and because of their interest in that sport. By being asked to take on other roles (e.g., being involved in the organization of the club, coaching others) the person may develop new strengths or discover preexisting strengths that they were not aware of. It is not uncommon for a spiral of clients satisfying multiple primary goods and developing multiple strengths, which can be described as an upward spiral or positive dynamic.

6.6 Conclusion

This chapter explored the application of the GLM in structuring supervision for individuals on parole or probation, including an illustration of how a human rights and social work perspective, using the framework of strengths-based practice (SBP) (Simmons et al., 2016) may serve as a guide to move through the three stages of the GLM: assessment, developing a GLP, and therapy. Each stage included an overview of eight principles based on the SBP: goal-oriented, strengths-oriented, context-oriented, hope-oriented, needs-oriented, therapeutic relationship, trauma-sensitive, and future-oriented. This approach supports a focus on well-being while working on relapse prevention and risk reduction. It aligns well with the GLM as a theoretical and practical framework for (community-based) forensic social work and mental health care.

This chapter highlighted some good practices and examples of community interventions throughout these stages. These can inspire clinicians and their community services in implementing the GLM. An important lesson is to use the methods that are already in one's therapeutic toolbox: the main challenge is how to apply these to support clients to fulfill their primary goods. Unlike a narrow, structured checklist approach, the GLM provides a broad guide that can be applied in different ways. Of course, structured tools can (and for some purposes should) be used. Thus, risk assessment should be done through the risk assessment tools provided for that purpose. Just as the mapping table can be used to better understand the primary goods associated with these risks, in order to treat them as well.

To monitor and review the most important aspects of implementing the GLM, practitioners may use the GLM fidelity monitoring tool (FID) (Prescott et al., 2022; see Chap. 4). This tool is designed to support GLM implementation when working with adult clients across forensic or correctional treatment settings. The tool is created for supervisory staff who are reviewing sessions, examining fundamental considerations and processes, as well as the GLM content. It also consists of a list of considerations to help support ongoing GLM implementation.

The different stages of implementing the GLM are dynamic. Effective implementation requires therapist and a service training, supervision and peer consultation. In Belgium, an initiative of the Department of Special Needs Education (Ghent University) and Forensisch Ambulant Begeleidingsteam (CAW Oost-Vlaanderen) developed a GLM network. Thematic GLM sessions are organized subsequent to an annual three-day GLM workshop led by Tony Ward and Mary Barnao that introduces participants to the implementation of the GLM in practice. These workshops provide a forum for practitioners, policymakers, and researchers to present and discuss their work or a particular GLM-related topic with other GLM network members. Core values and constructs of the SBP—such as resilience, hope, empowerment, self-determination, client involvement, person-in-environment (Franklin, 2015; Simmons et al., 2016, 2021)—are essential to sharing these good practices.

References

Ainsworth, M. D., Blehar, M. C., Waters, E., & Wall, S. (1978). *Patterns of attachment: A psychological study of the strange situation*. Erlbaum.
Baim, C., Brookes, S., & Mountford, A. (2002). *The geese theatre handbook : Drama with offenders and people at risk*. Waterside Press.
Baim, C., & Morrison, T. (2011). *Attachment-based practice with adults: Understanding strategies and promoting positive change*. Pavilion.
Barnao, M. (2013). The good lives model tool kit for mentally disordered offenders. *The Journal of Forensic Practice, 15*(3), 157–170.
Barnao, M., Ward, T., & Robertson, P. (2015). The good lives model: A new paradigm for forensic mental health. *Psychiatry, Psychology and Law, 23*(2), 288–301.
Borowski, A. (2022). On human dignity and social work. *The British Journal of Social Work, 52*(2), 609–623.
Bouverne-De Bie, M. (2002). Historische en actuele ontwikkelingen in de relatie tussen strafuitvoering en hulpverlening. In *Handboek Forensisch Welzijnswerk* (pp. 275–298). Academia Press.
Burlingame, G. M., & Jensen. (2017). Small group process and outcome research highlights: A 25-year perspective. *International Journal of Group Psychotherapy, 67*(2), 194–218.
Cantürk, M., Faraji, H., & Tezcan, A. E. (2021). The relationship between childhood traumas and crime in male prisoners. *Alpha Psychiatry, 22*(1), 56–60.
de Vogel, V., de Ruiter, C., Bouman, Y., & de Vries Robbé, M. (2012). *SAPROF. Guidelines for the assessment of protective factors for violence risk* (2nd ed.). Forum Educatief.
de Vries Robbé, M., Mann, R. E., Maruna, S., & Thornton, D. (2015). An exploration of protective factors supporting desistance from sexual offending. *Sexual Abuse, 27*(1), 16–33.
Doran, G. T. (1981). There's a S.M.A.R.T. way to write management's goals and objectives. *Management Review, 70*, 35–36.
Douglas, E. M., McCarthy, S. C., & Serino, P. A. (2014). Does a social work degree predict practice orientation? Measuring strengths-based practice among child welfare workers with the strengths-based practices inventory–provider version. *Journal of Social Work Education, 50*(2), 219–233.
Edwards, D., & Parkinson, K. (2018). *Family group conferences in social work: Involving families in social care decision making*. Policy Press.
Fenton, J. (2013). Risk aversion and anxiety in Scottish criminal justice social work: Can desistance and human rights agendas have an impact? *The Howard Journal of Criminal Justice, 52*(1), 77–90.
Fernandez, Y., Harris, A. J. R., Hanson, R. K., & Sparks, J. (2014). *STABLE-2007 coding manual* (Rev. ed.). Public Safety Canada.
Franklin, C. (2015). An update on strengths-based, solution-focused brief therapy. *Health & Social Work, 40*(2), 73–76.
Fortune, C. A., Ward, T., & Print, B. (2014). Integrating the good lives model with relapse prevention: Working with juvenile sex offenders. In D. Bromberg & W. O'Donohue (Eds.), *Toolkit for working with juvenile sex offenders* (pp. 405–426). Academic Press.
Fox, A., & Freestone, M. (2008). *Good lives and development (GLAD) on the Westgate unit: An evaluation of a new incentive scheme*. HM Prison Service.
Garrett, P. M. (2024). Human rights and social work: Making the case for human rights plus (hr+). *The British Journal of Social Work, 54*(5), 2107–2123.
Giulini, P., Emiletti, L., Garbarino, F., Scotti, A., Bradford, J. M., Looman, J., Saleh, F. M., & Brodsky, D. J. (2020). The treatment of sex offenders: An international perspective. In F. M. Saleh, J. M. Bradford, & D. J. Brodsky (Eds.), *Sex offenders: Identification, risk assessment, treatment, and legal issues* (2nd ed., pp. 391–418). Oxford University Press.
Grady, M. D., Levenson, J. S., Glover, J., Kavanagh, S., & Carter, K. (2022). "Hurt People Hurt Other People": The link between past trauma and sexual offending. *Sexual Offending: Theory, Research, and Prevention, 17*(1), 1–28.

Gxubane, T. (2016). The prospects of family group conferencing with youth sex offenders and their victims in South Africa. In T. Gavrielides (Ed.), *Offenders no more: An interdisciplinary restorative justice dialogue* (pp. 267–287). Nova Publishers.

Haight, B. K., Barba, B. E., Courts, N. F., & Tesh, A. S. (2002). Thriving: A life span theory. *Journal of Gerontological Nursing, 28*(3), 14–22.

Harlow, C. W. (1999). *Prior abuse reported by inmates and probationers*. U.S. Department of Justice.

Harris, D. A., & Levenson, J. S. (2020). Life on "the List" is a life lived in fear: Post-conviction traumatic stress in men convicted of sexual offenses. *International Journal of Offender Therapy and Comparative Criminology, 65*(6–7), 763–789.

Levenson, J. (2014). Incorporating trauma-informed care into evidence-based sex offender treatment. *Journal of Sexual Aggression, 20*(1), 9–22.

Levenson, J. S., Willis, G., & Prescott, D. (2016). Adverse childhood experiences in the lives of male sex offenders: Implications for trauma-informed care. *Sexual Abuse, 28*(4), 340–359.

Levenson, J. S., Willis, G., & Prescott, D. (2017). *Trauma-informed care: Transforming treatment for people who sexually abuse*. Safer Society Press.

Locke, E. A., & Latham, G. P. (2002). Building a practically useful theory of goal setting and task motivation: A 35-year odyssey. *American Psychologist, 57*(9), 705–717.

Mann, R. E., Webster, S. D., Schofield, C., & Marshall, W. L. (2004). Approach versus avoidance goals in relapse prevention with sexual offenders. *Sexual Abuse, 16*(1), 65–75.

Manthey, T., Knowles, B., Asher, D., & Wahab, S. (2011). Strengths-based practice and motivational interviewing. *Advances in Social Work, 12*, 126–151.

Marshall, W. L., Anderson, D., & Fernandez, Y. (1999). *Cognitive Behavioural treatment of sexual offenders*. Wiley.

Marshall, W. L., Marshall, L. E., Serran, G. A., & O'Brien, M. D. (2011). *Rehabilitating sexual offenders: A strength-based approach*. American Psychological Association.

Mehr, S. A., Singh, M., Knox, D., Ketter, D. M., Pickens-Jones, D., Atwood, S., Lucas, C., Jacoby, N., Egner, A. A., Hopkins, E. J., Howard, R. M., Hartshorne, J. K., Jennings, M. V., Simson, J., Bainbridge, C. M., Pinker, S., O'Donnell, T. J., Krasnow, M. M., & Glowacki, L. (2019). Universality and diversity in human song. *Science, 366*(6468), 1–17.

Messina, N., Grella, C., Burdon, W., & Prendergast, M. (2007). Childhood adverse events and current traumatic distress a comparison of men and women drug-dependent prisoners. *Criminal Justice and Behavior, 34*, 1385–1401.

Meyvis, W., Roose, R., & Vander Laenen, F. (2012). Van private reclassering naar maatschappelijke dienstverlening aan justitiecliënteel. In R. Roose, M. Bouverne-De Bie, K. Kloeck, W. Meyvis, & J. Vanacker (Eds.), *Handboek forensisch welzijnswerk: Ontwikkeling, beleid, organisatie & praktijk* (pp. 27–46). Academia Press.

Munninghoff, X. (2021). De Weg naar een Goed Leven. Een behandel methodiek voor adolescenten die seksueel grensoverschrijdend gedrag plegen. In *Presentation at GLM Session #3 (Slideshow)*. GLM Network.

Murray, K., & Hick, S. (2012). Structural social work. In M. Gray & S. Webb (Eds.), *Social work theories and methods* (pp. 273–287). Sage Publications.

Naessens, L. (2023). *Forensic social work : A human rights perspective*. University of Antwerp, Faculty of Social Sciences, Department of Sociology.

Prescott, D. S., & Levenson, J. S. (in press). Exploring trauma-informed care in a high-intensity program. In N. Blagden, B. Winder, K. Hocken, R. Lievesley, C. Harper, H. Swaby, & P. Banyard (Eds.), *Sexual cime & community (re)integration*. Palgrave.

Prescott, D. S., Willis, G. M., & Ward, T. (2022). Monitoring therapist fidelity to the good lives model (GLM). *International Journal of Offender Therapy and Comparative Criminology., 68*, 131. https://doi.org/10.1177/0306624X221086572

Purvis, M., Ward, T., & Willis, G. (2011). The good lives model in practice: Offense pathways and case management. *European Journal of Probation, 3*(2), 4–28.

Rapp, C. A., & Goscha, R. J. (2006). *The strengths model case management with psychiatric disabilities* (2nd ed.). Oxford University Press.

Rapp, C. A., Saleebey, D., & Sullivan, W. P. (2005). The future of strengths-based social work. *Advances in Social Work, 6*(1), 79–90.

Ross, E. C., Polascheck, D. L. L., & Ward, T. (2008). The therapeutic alliance: A theoretical revision for offender rehabilitation. *Aggression and Violent Behavior, 13*(6), 462–480.

Saleebey, D. (Ed.). (2006). *The strengths perspective in social work practice* (4th ed.). Pearson Education, Inc.

Simmons, C. A., Shapiro, V. B., Accomazzo, S., & Manthey, T. J. (2016). Strengths-based social work: A social work metatheory to guide the profession. In N. Coady & P. Lehmann (Eds.), *Theoretical perspectives for direct social work practice* (3rd ed., pp. 130–152). Springer.

Simmons, C. A., Shapiro, V. B., Accomazzo, S., & Manthey, T. J. (2021). Strengths-based practice: A metatheory to guide the social work profession. In K. W. Bolton, J. C. Hall, & P. Lehmann (Eds.), *Theoretical perspectives for direct social work practice: A generalist-eclectic approach* (4th ed., pp. 100–115). Springer. Retrieved from https://escholarship.org/content/qt1p44c8cs/qt1p44c8cs.pdf. Accessed December 19, 2024

Snyder, C. R., Harris, C., Anderson, J. R., Holleran, S. A., Irving, L. M., Sigmon, S. T., Yoshinobu, L., Gibb, J., Langelle, C., & Harney, P. (1991). The will and the ways: Development and validation of an individual-differences measure of hope. *Journal of Personality and Social Psychology, 60*(4), 570–585.

Snyder, C. R., Rand, K. L., & Sigmon, D. R. (2018). Hope theory: A member of the positive psychology family. In M. W. Gallagher & S. J. Lopez (Eds.), *The Oxford handbook of hope* (pp. 27–43). Oxford University Press.

Taylor, A., & Frost, A. (2017). Social work and the justice system. In M. Connolly, L. Harms, & J. Maidment (Eds.), *Social work contexts and practice* (4th ed., pp. 235–249). Oxford University Press.

Van Garsse, L. (2012). Achtergronden van een complexe bevoegdheidsverkaveling. In R. Roose, M. Bouverne-De Bie, K. Kloeck, W. Meyvis, & J. Vanacker (Eds.), *Handboek forensisch welzijnswerk: ontwikkeling, beleid, organisatie & praktijk* (pp. 93–103). Academia Press.

Verellen, R., & De Boeck, M. (2020). Het samenwerkingsakkoord vertaald naar een traject voor de begeleiding en behandeling van daders van seksueel misbruik in Vlaanderen. In K. Goethals, M. De Boeck, T. Dilliën, W. Huys, & A. Nuyts (Eds.), *Handboek behandeling van seksueel afwijkend gedrag* (pp. 39–66). Gompel & Svacina.

Versweyvelt, A.-S., Put, J., Opgenhaffen, T., & Van der Straete, I. (2018). *Beroepsgeheim en hulpverlening*. die Keure.

Wanzeele, W., & Oltenfreiter, S. (2020). De zoektocht naar een behandelkader dat werkt: wat kunnen we leren van de Risk-Need-Responsivity principes en het Good Lives Model? In K. Goethals, M. De Boeck, T. Dilliën, W. Huys, & A. Nuyts (Eds.), *Handboek behandeling van seksueel afwijkend gedrag* (pp. 203–233). Gompel & Svacina.

Wanzeele, W., & Severs, K. (2020). Good lives music. In *Presentation at GLM session #2 (slideshow)*. GLM Network.

Ward, T. (2009). Dignity and human rights in correctional practice. *European Journal of Probation, 1*(2), 112–127.

Ward, T. (2011). Human rights and dignity in offender rehabilitation. *Journal of Forensic Psychology Practice, 11*(2–3), 103–123.

Ward, T., & Brown, M. (2004). The good lives model and conceptual issues in offender rehabilitation. *Psychology, Crime & Law, 10*(3), 243–257.

Ward, T., Mann, R. E., & Gannon, T. A. (2007). The good lives model of offender rehabilitation: Clinical implications. *Aggression and Violent Behavior, 12*(1), 87–107.

Ward, T., Vess, J., Collie, R. M., & Gannon, T. A. (2006). Risk management or goods promotion: The relationship between approach and avoidance goals in treatment for sex offenders. *Aggression and Violent Behavior, 11*(4), 378–393.

Willis, G. M., & Ward, T. (2024). Evidence for the good lives model in supporting rehabilitation and desistance from offending. In L. A. Craig, L. Dixon, & T. A. Gannon (Eds.), *The Wiley handbook of what works in correctional rehabilitation: An evidence-based approach to theory, assessment and treatment* (2nd ed.). Wiley-Blackwell.

Wood, F. (2015). Working with personality disordered offenders; responsivity issues and management strategies. *Prison Service Journal, 218*, 24–30.

Yates, P. M. (2009). Using the good lives model to motivate sexual offenders to participate in treatment. In D. S. Prescott (Ed.), *Building motivation for change in sexual offenders* (pp. 74–95). Safer Society Press.

Yates, P., Prescott, D. S., & Ward, T. (2010). *Applying the good lives and self-regulation models to sex offender treatment: A practical guide for clinicians*. Safer Society Press.

Chapter 7
Forensic Mental Health

7.1 Introduction

Most practitioners working in forensic mental health services would agree that rehabilitating individuals with mental disorders who have offended (IMDO)[1] is an inherently complex process, although it can also be rewarding. Forensic service users (FSUs) commonly present with a diverse set of rehabilitative needs, including serious offending, often of a violent or sexual nature (Rutherford & Duggan, 2008); chronic and comorbid psychiatric disorders (Palijan et al., 2010); cognitive impairments (Fioravanti et al., 2012); and histories of severe trauma, especially maltreatment in childhood (Spitzer et al., 2006).

FSUs commonly have complex motivational issues that make it difficult to engage them in rehabilitation. These motivational issues may relate to the individuals themselves (e.g., difficulty trusting authority figures) or to the clinical context and therapeutic climate in which rehabilitation is provided (Hodge & Renswick, 2002). Admission to forensic mental health services is usually involuntary and involves legally mandated treatment with outcomes intended to benefit society as much, if not more than the client. Importantly, direct and indirect coercion can undermine treatment motivation, disrupt the therapeutic process in general, and negatively impact the well-being of IMDOs (Lutz et al., 2022).

Adding to the challenges of forensic rehabilitation is the balancing act that practitioners are required to perform, providing treatment and care for IMDOs at the same time they are tasked with protecting society by reducing recidivism. Often, practitioners must effectively function as double agents, simultaneously helping clients and being agents of social control (Blackburn, 2004). However, these dual

[1] The use of this term is intended to draw attention to the fact that IMDOs are, first and foremost, people who are not defined by their mental illness and offending.

T. Ward et al., *The Good Lives Model of Correctional Rehabilitation*,
Advances in Preventing and Treating Violence and Aggression,
https://doi.org/10.1007/978-3-031-95559-4_7

responsibilities can pull practitioners in opposing directions that may not be easily reconciled, particularly in more complex cases (Ward, 2013). This can create ethical flashpoints in forensic teams where issues such as leave applications, treatment priorities, and the management of risky behavior may be hotly debated.

The challenge of forensic rehabilitation is typically undertaken in a complex institutional environment, shaped by a raft of legal and organizational imperatives, with a strong emphasis on custody and widespread restrictions on liberty. While the restrictive features of forensic mental health services are often predicated on concerns about risk, they can jeopardize recovery, undermine agency, and lead service users to feel dehumanized, dissatisfied with care, and powerless (Barnao & Ward, 2015; Chow & Priebe, 2013). In some cases, periods of incarceration may lead to institutionalization, which can have harmful impacts, including loss of independence, responsibility, and identity, and identifying as one of the sick (Chow & Priebe, 2013). Thus, the context in which forensic care is delivered can compound FSU's suffering and problems and amplify the difficulties that practitioners face in rehabilitating them.

The complexity of forensic practice requires comprehensive theories to help practitioners navigate the clinical, ethical, and conceptual challenges that arise when working with FSUs. Ward and Durrant's (2021) recent formulation of a practice framework encapsulates the broad and integrative type of theory that could help to guide all aspects of forensic rehabilitation. As outlined in Chap. 1, a practice theory sets out the overarching values, principles, aims, and etiological assumptions used to guide interventions and helps practitioners translate these principles into practice. Practice theories are essentially hybrid theories, containing a blend of normative, knowledge, and practice elements. They can be distinguished from treatment theories, which are more specific in nature, and involve the application of principles and practical strategies to change an aspect of a person's behavior.

To date, this type of overarching framework has received little attention in the published forensic mental health literature (Robertson et al., 2011). This chapter posits that the GLM, when adapted for use with individuals with mental disorder, has the potential to fill this theoretical void in forensic mental health and to provide an integrative and comprehensive framework to guide practitioners in all aspects of their work.

This chapter will demonstrate how GLM has promising implications for FSUs. While the traditional approach to forensic rehabilitation has limitations, using the GLM in a forensic mental health context can enhance the way in which rehabilitation is delivered. An enriched form of the GLM can be used with individuals who have offended and who also experience mental health issues. A case study will illustrate how the GLM can promote a more cohesive approach to forensic rehabilitation that helps to engage service users.

7.2 The Traditional Approach to Forensic Rehabilitation

Describing the usual approach to rehabilitating FSUs is a thorny task since the focus, in the forensic mental health treatment literature, has tended to be on the application and evaluation of specific interventions rather than on rehabilitation programs as a whole (Barnao & Ward, 2015). Consequently, many important questions remain unanswered. For example, what are the aims of these programs? What types of interventions are typically included and how are they selected? What theoretical frameworks underpin the interventions that are employed? And how well equipped are these theoretical frameworks to assist practitioners in rehabilitating FSUs?

Barnao and Ward's (2015) review of the published literature on interventions in forensic mental health shed some light on these important questions. Categorizing treatments according to their broad theoretical orientation, they identified three paradigms that underpinned most of the treatments reported in the forensic mental health literature over the previous 15 years. The first of these, which encompassed the bulk of the forensic intervention literature, was a mental health paradigm that focuses on treating mental disorder, alleviating suffering, and improving psychological and social functioning. This category encompassed a range of treatments "imported" from the general mental health literature such as: the use of psychopharmacology; illness education programs; dialectic behavior therapy, schema therapy, eye movement desensitization and reprocessing (EMDR); and group programs based on a cognitive behavior therapy (CBT) approach (e.g., anger management, problem-solving skills).

The second paradigm that Barnao and Ward (2015) identified, which accounted for the second highest volume of literature, was risk management. Literature categorized according to this broad theoretical orientation is primarily concerned with protecting the community through reducing an individual's risk of recidivism. Derived from the offender rehabilitation literature, the programs reported in the forensic mental health treatment literature were largely based on Andrews and Bonta's risk-need-responsivity (RNR) model of offender rehabilitation (Andrews et al., 1990; Andrews & Bonta, 2010) and included offender behavior programs such as reasoning and rehabilitation (R&R; Ross & Fabiano, 1985) and enhanced thinking skills (ETS; Clark, 2000).

A third perspective, accounting for an exceedingly small proportion of the intervention literature, was the strength-based approach. This type of approach represents a fundamental shift in perspective from the two theoretical orientations outlined above (i.e., mental health and risk management), transcending a focus on problems and deficits to take a more holistic view of individuals, including consideration of their strengths, personal priorities, and hopes. One of the best-known strength-based approaches, which was first used in general mental health services, is the recovery model. Founded on the principles of hope, empowerment, healing, and connection (Jacobson & Greenley, 2001), it promotes patient choice, responsibility, and self-determination (Pouncey & Lukens, 2010). Another example of a strength-based approach is the good lives model (GLM; Ward & Maruna, 2007;

Ward & Stewart, 2003) which, over the past decade or so, has been further developed for use in a forensic mental health context (Barnao et al., 2010; Barnao et al., 2015).

Barnao and Ward (2015) found that, in order to cater to IMDOs' wide-ranging therapeutic needs, standard forensic rehabilitation programs combined a mixture of interventions derived from the mental health and risk management perspectives. The resulting blended rehabilitation programs typically included a mixture of therapeutic ingredients, such as psychotropic medication, trauma interventions, and offender behavior programs, which were selected according to individual clients' specific problems and diagnoses (e.g., Hodgins, 2002; Rice & Harris, 1997). Strength-based interventions and approaches, including implementation of recovery philosophy and principles, were sometimes also incorporated into programs alongside interventions targeting risk and mental health issues.

Some general inferences can be made about the nature of forensic rehabilitation programs. First, the primary objectives of forensic rehabilitation appear to be to treat mental illness and other clinical needs, and to reduce the risk of reoffending. Second, rehabilitation programs combine a variety of interventions derived from mental health and risk management paradigms to achieve these dual objectives. Third, these interventions are selected using an actuarial approach, which involves the straightforward application of the most effective treatment known for a particular problem or disorder. Fourth, this method of treatment selection, which has been explicitly recommended by some authors (e.g., Hodgins, 2002; Rice & Harris, 1997), reflects the unavailability, until very recently, of broad rehabilitation theories and practice frameworks to guide intervention planning.

So how well equipped is the standard type of forensic program to rehabilitate FSUs? In short, such programs have some real weaknesses that can undermine effective rehabilitation. The most fundamental problem with an approach based on the mental health/risk management hybrid is that it fails to provide a cohesive theoretical basis for understanding IMDOs and their core rehabilitation needs. The issue is that the constituent theoretical frameworks in this uneasy amalgam contain different values and principles, rehabilitation aims, etiological theories, and ways of approaching intervention that, when combined, potentially raise more issues than they solve.

A further difficulty with blended approaches is that they do not provide clinicians with sufficient guidance on the importance that should be placed on addressing criminogenic needs versus treating mental disorder. Although mental disorder may be conceived of as a criminogenic need when it is implicated in offending, (e.g., in the case of psychotically driven violence), blended approaches provide little direction on treatment priorities in cases where mental illness is not etiologically related to offending, or when other comorbid mental health conditions are present (as is commonly the case). In addition, they fail to provide guidance on the priority that should be given to addressing other issues that do not directly address mental illness or risk but are intended to improve quality of life and/or promote strengths.

Further problems arise from the way in which treatment decision-making is approached in traditional forensic rehabilitation programs. Specifically, the use of an actuarial approach is not well suited to forensic practice because there is no direct or clear link between key problems, such as violence, and treatment (Hart et al., 2011). Selecting interventions according to an individual's specific problems and disorders creates a real risk that rehabilitation planning will be undertaken in a fragmented, unsystematic, and mechanical manner that overlooks the core issues underpinning the IMDO's difficulties and, indeed, the person themselves (Barnao et al., 2010; Barnao, Ward, & Casey, 2016; Barnao, Ward, & Robertson, 2016).

Finally, forensic programs that are underpinned by a mental health/risk hybrid tend to be deficit-focused and typically lead to a preponderance of avoidant treatment goals (i.e., goals that are centered on the elimination of unwanted symptoms and the avoidance of negative consequences). The problem is that IMDOs may have little motivation to engage in rehabilitation programs that emphasize avoidance goals, particularly when these goals are not linked to their important values and aspirations (Ward et al., 2007). The deficit-focused nature of these programs may also undermine the therapeutic alliance, which is a serious problem given the demonstrated link between therapeutic relationships, treatment outcomes (Ackerman & Hilsenroth, 2003; Leach, 2005), and FSU satisfaction (e.g., Bressington et al., 2011).

To summarize, the traditional approach to forensic rehabilitation has some major weaknesses which arise from the practice of blending antagonistic theoretical frameworks (mental health and RNR) and aspects of the constituent models themselves (e.g., deficit-focused, focus on avoidance goals). Crucially, these weaknesses may undermine effective rehabilitation and obscure what should be clearly in focus: the client as a person.

The findings of a qualitative study that explored detained FSUs' perceptions of their rehabilitation (Barnao et al., 2015) provide empirical support for the problems associated with orthodox forensic programs. The participants described an inconsistent and uncoordinated approach to their care, confusion about their rehabilitation pathways, relationships with staff that were of variable quality, and an overall lack of person-centered care. In addition, they considered that there was a disproportionate emphasis on their mental illness, which prevented them from being seen as people. These perceptions of the rehabilitation landscape were reflected in the participants' self-evaluations, which were underdeveloped and deficit-focused, and in their profound sense of powerlessness. Significantly, the participants' representations of their care suggested a mixture of assessments, interventions, and paradigms that did not fit well, and a strong emphasis on a biologically oriented psychiatric model. Barnao et al. (2015) posited that the heart of the problem was the absence of a superordinate rehabilitation framework to integrate the various elements of forensic practice.

A survey of more recent literature on interventions in forensic mental health suggests that there have been some significant developments since Barnao & Ward's, 2015 review, such as the increased use of third wave therapies (e.g., mindfulness, ACT, compassion-focused therapy) and the more widespread application of recovery-oriented principles in forensic practice (Simpson & Penney, 2018). However, what has not changed in the intervening years is the paucity of research on broad theories and practice frameworks to guide forensic rehabilitation.

7.3 What the GLM Can Offer Forensic Mental Health

The GLM is an overarching model of offender rehabilitation that has the potential to address many of the weaknesses of traditional forensic rehabilitation programs. When augmented for use with forensic populations, it can provide a comprehensive practice framework to assist practitioners weave together all the different threads of forensic rehabilitation. The GLM allows practitioners to develop, in collaboration with FSUs, a single, theoretically driven case formulation that explains an individual's offending and other problems and helps to identify the core issues that need to be addressed in their rehabilitation. More specific treatment models and theories (e.g., CBT, DBT, attachment theory) and different perspectives (e.g., risk management, mental health, recovery) can be integrated within the GLM framework. Indeed, the dual aims of the GLM—to enhance individuals' well-being while reducing their risk of further offending—brings these different perspectives together and may help forensic practitioners bypass the ethical tensions inherent in the care of the person versus societal protection dichotomy associated with blended approaches. It works because, in the GLM, these two aims are synergistic: a core assumption of the GLM is that the most effective way to create a safer society is to help individuals to develop more fulfilling, socially integrated lives. Another attractive feature of the GLM is that it combines direction about what should be accomplished in an individual's rehabilitation with explicit guidance on how rehabilitation should be delivered, thereby linking the content and process of intervention. Critical aspects of the rehabilitation process—such as the therapeutic relationship, motivational issues, matters of ethics and human rights, and the broader treatment context—are specifically addressed in the GLM.

In addition to promoting a more cohesive approach to forensic rehabilitation, there are several other reasons why the GLM may be particularly well suited for use with FSUs. First, its strong emphasis on human agency (e.g., Ward et al., 2007), outlined in Chap. 1, is particularly germane to the highly disempowered population of IMDOs. The GLM holds that clients, like other human beings, are self-determining agents who actively seek to satisfy their life values (i.e., primary goods) through whatever means are available to them. This assumption also applies, with some caveats, to IMDOs; however, mental illness, the imposition of court-ordered restrictions on liberty, and aspects of service provision can strip a person of their agency. Crucially, when employed as the overarching framework for forensic rehabilitation, the GLM can foster the restoration of human agency through its emphasis on developing and enacting a person-centered good life plan (i.e., plan for living) in a spirit of collaboration and respect.

The GLM can also assist IMDOs to move away from a problem-focused view of themselves and to establish a new personal or practical identity The GLM posits that an individual's prioritized primary goods are embedded within specific roles or activities. For example, a person for whom relationships are important may place value on being a loving partner or a responsive parent. Identifying a person's core practical identities, along with their associated primary goods and goals, is crucial for effective intervention planning since these elements are placed at the very center of the individual's good life plan. This comprehensive life plan, which revolves around the individual's core goals and practical identities, also specifies the internal and external conditions that are required for the person to achieve their aspirations. Importantly, the GLM's strong focus on the promotion of a positive self-identity, which reflects the person's most cherished values and goals, is highly germane to the forensic population. Previous research has indicated that the self-evaluations of FSUs tend to be deficit-focused, with an emphasis on their mental illness and offending (Barnao et al., 2015).

Another reason why the GLM may be a good fit for forensic mental health services is that it is sensitive to diversity, including cultural diversity. In fact, the GLM is not only equipped to include culture and other person-specific characteristics in intervention but it requires their inclusion, according to the wishes of the client. This is an important consideration when defining practice frameworks for FSUs, given the overrepresentation of ethnic minorities and indigenous people in forensic mental health services (McKenna, 2020) and the importance of using interventions and models that resonate with these populations. As a framework that recognizes individual differences in what constitutes a good life for different people, the GLM provides practitioners with the flexibility to tailor rehabilitation according to the needs of the individual and their community. It recognizes that culture can influence what constitutes a good life and the ways in which individuals seek primary goods, yet it does not make assumptions about an individual's similarities or differences to their cultural group or prescribe a set of values for clients (Leaming & Willis, 2016).

Drawing on the sociocultural context of Aoteoroa-New Zealand, several researchers have highlighted the convergence of Māori (indigenous) models, such as *Te Whare Tapa Whā*, and the GLM, noting such parallels as their holistic approach, their emphasis on prudential values (or human goods) in understanding offending and informing interventions, their view of clients as having equal moral status to non-offending individuals, their focus on individual strengths and capacities, and their view of offending as an issue of both well-being and a social problem (Leaming & Willis, 2016; Strauss-Hughes et al., 2022). Furthermore, both the GLM and Māori perspectives conceptualize offending as a symptom of a deeper underlying problem, and both are equipped to view colonization and discriminatory sociocultural contexts as playing a key causal role in offending behavior (Strauss-Hughes et al., 2022). The crucial point is that the GLM and indigenous models, such as *Te Whare Tapa Whā,* are highly compatible and can provide complementary perspectives that allow for a richer understanding of the person.

Finally, there is reason to believe that the GLM—through its attention to the individual's life values, goals, and strengths—may be more appealing to FSUs than the more traditional, deficit-focused type of forensic rehabilitation program. Similar evidence suggests that integrating the GLM into interventions for individuals who have offended has the potential to enhance treatment engagement, reduce dropout rates, and result in better outcomes (e.g., Simons et al., 2006). Other research exploring the application of the GLM to IMDOs suggests that the GLM can enhance the experience of forensic rehabilitation from the service user perspective (Barnao,

Ward, & Casey, 2016; Barnao, Ward, & Robertson, 2016) and play a key role in promoting treatment engagement (Gannon et al., 2011).

7.4 Application of the GLM to Forensic Mental Health

Despite its potential as a rehabilitation framework for forensic mental health, the GLM has been largely overlooked by practitioners working in this specialty (see Barnao et al., 2010; Gannon et al., 2011; Barnao, Ward, & Casey, 2016; Barnao, Ward, & Robertson, 2016; Byrne, 2020 for exceptions). One likely reason is that applying the GLM to individuals who have a history of offending and ongoing mental illness requires some theoretical augmentation of the model.

Mental illness fits within the assumptions of the GLM, specifically on three key points. The first of these pertains to the way mental illness negatively impacts an individual's ability to satisfy primary goods. The second concerns the way psychiatric symptomatology can sometimes function as a means by which primary goods are sought. Finally, the third relates to the key role of mental health service provision in facilitating or obstructing an individual's capacity to satisfy primary goods.

7.4.1 Impact of Mental Illness on Individual's Ability to Satisfy Primary Human Goods

Disturbance to mental health inevitably compromises a person's capacity to satisfy primary goods. Mental health problems undermine the personal competencies and skills required to fulfill a range of human needs. For example, a person who is depressed may withdraw from friends and family, have little interest in previously enjoyed activities, experience debilitating fatigue, struggle to concentrate, and engage in negative rumination, among other symptoms. Consequently, the person may lose their sense of connection with loved ones, stop engaging in leisure pursuits and community activities, be unable to perform their job effectively, and experience a sense of unhappiness and emotional turmoil. Using the terminology of the GLM, the person's capacity to satisfy human goods such as relationships, play, community, work, happiness, peace of mind, and agency has been hindered by their symptoms of depression. The deficit this creates in the person's lifestyle (i.e., problems with scope) is likely to further undermine their mental well-being, since the absence of primary goods is related to psychological problems of various kinds (Emmons, 1999; Ward & Maruna, 2007).

The discussion this far has focused on the way that symptoms of mental illness can undermine an individual's ability to satisfy important life goals. In the GLM, these types of obstacles are referred to as problems with internal capacity. However, environmental factors associated with mental illness can also act as barriers to a person being able to satisfy human goods, signifying problems with external capacity. For example, a person suffering from depression may experience financial hardship arising from an extended absence from work or the loss of their job. This, in turn, may limit opportunities to engage in social and recreational activities and even result in difficulties accessing the necessities of life, such as adequate food, heating, and medical care (i.e., impede access to primary goods such as play, relationships, and life).

This example illustrates how mental illness can compromise an individual's quality of life by creating problems with personal capacity and restricting the opportunities, resources, and support that are available to them in their environment. These problems may be temporary, with the capacity to access human goods being restored as the person recovers. They can also be more pervasive and enduring, as in the case of severe and chronic mental illness. Since this chapter is concerned with the application of the GLM to FSUs, the discussion that follows will focus on the most severe forms of mental illness, such as schizophrenia, which often characterize this population.

What is clear from the research literature is that individuals who suffer from severe mental health difficulties face an array of challenges to satisfying human goods. For example, mental illness is associated with higher rates of serious physical health problems and premature mortality. It may lead people into poverty and homelessness, and it can create vulnerability to abuse and neglect (World Health Organization [WHO], 2013). All of these problems create serious obstacles to fulfilling the primary good of life. In addition, early-onset mental disorders may prevent individuals from completing their education and successfully establishing themselves in careers, presenting barriers to the primary goods of knowledge and excellence in work. As one of the most important determinants of misery (Layard et al., 2013), mental disorder is also likely to curtail an individual's capacity to satisfy the primary goods of inner peace and happiness.

People who experience mental illness face many external obstacles to satisfying primary goods, including stigma and discrimination, which can be as limiting as the illness itself. Surveys of public attitudes toward people with mental illness continue to show high levels of fear, intolerance, and beliefs supportive of social exclusion, particularly when the individual has also carried out violent offenses (Brooker & Ullmann, 2008). Such attitudes impede social relationships, undermine community integration, and have been shown to adversely affect a person's ability to secure work, housing, and insurance (Corrigan, 2004). As such, they prevent individuals from accessing the primary goods of community, friendship, life, and excellence in work, among others.

One of the most devastating effects of severe mental illness and its sequelae is its capacity to undermine an individual's autonomy (i.e., the primary good of agency). One aspect of agency that may be compromised in individuals with major mental illness is the capacity to carry out self-directed, intentional actions in the service of achieving valued goals. In addition to undermining agency from the inside, severe mental disorder can lead to state-imposed restrictions on a person's liberty. For example, individuals adjudged to pose a danger to themselves or others may be detained against their will, subjected to compulsory treatment, and have their right to privacy overridden. Indeed, FSUs experience even more comprehensive encroachments on their freedom than those detained in prisons, since there is no time limit on their legally mandated detention and supervision. Some aspects of mental health service provision can further erode patient agency and thereby obstruct access to other primary goods. Importantly, when individuals' sense of agency is diminished, their ability to satisfy other human goods is restricted and their dignity undermined (Ward & Syversen, 2009).

7.4.2 Symptoms of Mental Illness as Secondary Goods

While mental illness can impede an individual's ability to satisfy universally sought-after goods, there are times when the symptoms of mental illness, and associated behaviors, may simultaneously provide the means by which valued primary goods are sought and, to some extent, attained. A few examples, drawn from clinical experience, will serve to illustrate this point.

Alfred, an elderly man with chronic schizophrenia who strangled his mother during an episode of psychosis, was an avid collector of educational books. Virtually every bit of floor space in his bedroom was covered with piles of hefty tomes, and staff at his supported accommodation were concerned that he would trip over them and hurt himself. While staff regarded Alfred's constant and secretive purchasing of books as symptomatic of a hoarding disorder, for Alfred ownership of the books represented the highly valued attribute of being educated (i.e., the primary good of knowledge). Alfred had been devastated when his university career was truncated by the early onset of schizophrenia but subsequently took comfort in surrounding himself with textbooks on a wide variety of subjects.

Peter, a middle-aged man with no previous history of offending, stabbed his mother to death while in the throes of psychosis. He attributed the homicide to having been poisoned at a restaurant he ate at shortly before the tragic event. This delusional belief proved to be intractable despite intensive therapy aimed at helping him to gain insight into his offending. Peter's delusion could be conceptualized as a way of absolving himself from an act that would otherwise have caused him profound anguish and called into question his perception of himself as a good man (i.e., an attempt to satisfy the primary good of inner peace).

Finally, the case of Mohammed, a young Muslim man with a delusional disorder, illustrates how psychotically driven behavior, including violence, can be conceptualized as an attempt to satisfy universally sought-after human goods, albeit within the context of an atypical way of viewing the world (Bentall, 2003). Mohammed assaulted his neighbor who he believed had inserted web cameras in his room to catch him watching pornography. His violence represented an attempt to stop the perceived invasion of his privacy (i.e., primary good of agency) and to alleviate the resulting feelings of anger and anxiety (i.e., primary good of inner peace). An exploration of Mohammed's background revealed that he had been displaced from his native country due to civil war and had subsequently spent 10 years living in a refugee camp. As a result of these experiences, Mohammed developed a sensitivity to issues of autonomy and privacy (i.e., primary good of agency), themes that were incorporated into his psychosis. This case example also highlights how psychosis can increase the salience of a primary good for an individual and, through its disinhibiting effect on behavior, influence the means by which the primary good is sought. Conceptualizing behaviors that are driven by mental disorder as concrete ways of pursuing human goods encourages practitioners to look beyond psychiatric symptoms and explore the goals that individuals are pursuing through their actions.

To summarize, mental illness can result in a variety of problems in an individual's way of life or good lives plan (GLP). First, it can undermine the internal and external capacities required to satisfy valued primary goods. Second, these problems with capacity can lead to a lack of scope in an individual's life, which can create further psychological problems and hinder recovery from mental illness. Third, the symptoms and behaviors associated with mental illness can represent a means of seeking out primary goods. As the case examples have illustrated, even individuals who have problems with reality testing are seeking to achieve some human goal(s). While their approach may be bizarre and/or socially unacceptable and their view of the world atypical, the underlying need(s) is legitimate and shared by all human beings. Finally, individuals who commit offenses when mentally unwell may experience a fourth type of problem in their GLP—a problem with conflict. Problems with conflict can arise when there is a clash between two primary goods that are sought. Conflict can sometimes also arise within the same good when there is a clash in the means used to attain it. To illustrate, consider the case of a devoted mother suffering from postpartum psychosis who committed infanticide in response to an altruistic delusion that she was saving her baby from a fate literally worse than death. Although the infanticide was motivated by love for her child (i.e., primary good of relationship), as her psychosis subsided her actions caused her profound anguish because of their utter dissonance with her usual means of pursuing the same value, which was to care for and protect her baby.

7.4.3 Service Provision as Facilitator of or Barrier to Primary Human Good Acquisition

According to the GLM, a key task of rehabilitation is to equip individuals with the environmental conditions and internal resources to obtain primary goods in prosocial and adaptive ways. Individuals suffering from severe mental illness are likely to experience deprivation across multiple areas of their life (e.g., financial hardship, housing problems, unemployment, social isolation), and these problems must be addressed if they are to have any chance of leading a fulfilling life.

Of course, equipping individuals with the external resources to satisfy important life goals is much more challenging when they are compulsorily detained, typically in institutional environments with high levels of security. These environments tend to be highly controlled and regimented, severely curtailing freedom of movement and choice, commonly restricting access to personal belongings and contact with loved ones, and prohibiting sexual intimacy. Furthermore, these restrictions can last for decades (Hare Duke et al., 2018).

Despite the immense challenges, it is possible for secure services to mitigate some of the organizational and legal constraints to individuals leading a fulfilling life and to actively foster activities, experiences, and relationships that promote access to human goods. For example, supportive relationships with staff can provide service users with a much-needed source of human connection, providing a means of satisfying the primary good of relationships. The importance of positive staff/client relationships is underscored by evidence indicating that psychiatric service users perceive the quality of the helping relationship as the most important factor for good care (Björkman et al., 1995; Johansson & Eklund, 2003). Similarly, communicating with service users in a transparent and respectful manner, taking their concerns seriously, and working collaboratively wherever possible to support their goals can help to promote a sense of self-determination (primary good of agency). In addition, making a selection of programs, interventions, and activities (e.g., vocational, recreational, educational, spiritual, cultural) available can allow service users to access a wide range of primary goods (e.g., excellence in work, excellence in play, knowledge, creativity, spirituality, community), and to prioritize those that are of particular importance to them.

However, "care" and "treatment" can unremittingly curtail incarcerated individuals' ability to satisfy human goods, particularly when it is provided in an institutional environment. Research describing psychiatric and FSUs' perceptions of care suggests that it may offer few opportunities for meaningful activity; devoid of genuine connections with staff; and even experienced as repressive, dehumanizing, and corrosive (e.g., Barnao et al., 2015; Farnworth et al., 2004; Hörberg et al., 2012; Lilja & Hellzen, 2008). Other studies have highlighted the negative effects of highly restrictive treatment environments on the quality of life of FSUs in inpatient facilities, especially with respect to depression and suicidality (Büsselmann et al., 2020; Franke et al., 2019).

A study of experiences of older IMDOs underscores the importance of environmental opportunities and support for incarcerated individuals and how they influence perceptions of care (De Smet et al., 2015). The study unexpectedly found that participants expressed more positive and less negative experiences in prison when compared to other institutional care settings (e.g., psychiatric hospitals and residential units for persons with an intellectual disability). The decisive factors in participants' more positive experiences of prison appeared to be the provision of activities, including paid work, and the availability and quality of psychosocial support. In contrast, individuals' negative experiences of institutional care were related to a lack of occupational activities, experiencing therapy as not useful, and a lack of personal attention.

Thus, the GLM reinforces that the quality and effectiveness of rehabilitation is inextricably linked to the wider context in which it is delivered and the degree to which it promotes access to human goods. As such, the care setting has profound implications for individuals' well-being, treatment motivation, recovery from mental illness, and consequently their recidivism risk.

The forensic version of the GLM has three aims: (1) to enhance the well-being of IMDOs by equipping them with the capacities to live a meaningful, healthy, and prosocial life; (2) to promote their recovery from mental illness; and (3) to protect the community by reducing their risk of recidivism. The following case example highlights how the GLM can assist practitioners to integrate these aims into a cohesive rehabilitation plan centered on what is most important to the individual.

7.5 Case Example

7.5.1 Background

Hemi, a 50-year-old, single man of mixed Māori and European ancestry, is a detained FSU with a diagnosis of schizophrenia and no prior history of offending. Following a frenzied attack on his mother whom he stabbed to death while psychotic, he was found not guilty of homicide by reason of insanity. He is the youngest of 12 siblings and until he was 13 was raised by his paternal grandparents, who were Māori. Hemi's grandparents lived in a remote coastal settlement in New Zealand, maintained regular contact with extended family living in the area, taught Hemi about his *whakapapa* (genealogy), and instilled in him a strong connection to his physical environment. The young Hemi spent his free time collecting shells and stones from which to make jewelry, painting landscapes and native birds, and helping his grandfather with his woodwork projects.

Sadly, Hemi's happy and secure life ended abruptly with his grandmother's sudden death followed, soon after, by a serious deterioration in his grandfather's health. The grief-stricken Hemi was subsequently transferred to the care of his parents, who lived in the city. Hemi found this transition extremely difficult, because he had not spent much time with his family, and their way of life was very different from everything he knew. He saw very little of his father, who worked long hours, and tried to avoid his mother whom he experienced as critical, controlling, and rejecting. He felt isolated from his older siblings, because they had been raised apart and had all left home. He struggled to fit in at his new school, and largely kept to himself. He was, however, an able student who excelled at woodwork and art.

On leaving school, he took up an apprenticeship as a builder but was forced to abandon his training after just a few months following a psychotic episode. Confined to home with little to occupy him, Hemi became increasingly apathetic, inactive, and socially isolated. He was often sullen and terse in his interactions with his mother and would forget to complete the chores she requested of him. Their relationship deteriorated further following the death of his father a few years later. He stopped taking his antipsychotic medication and became convinced that his mother was Jezebel, a biblical figure denounced as a murderer, and that she was planning to kill him.

7.5.2 GLM Case Formulation

In his psychotically driven violence Hemi was seeking to exert some control over his situation (i.e., primary good of agency), to take a preemptive strike at his mother who he believed posed a danger to him (i.e., primary good of life), and to assuage his fear of being harmed (i.e., primary good of peace of mind). Hemi's way of life at the time of his offending was problematic in several respects (i.e., there were several flaws in his GLP). Most obviously, his impoverished lifestyle was poorly aligned with his overarching primary goods of creativity and community, and he had little agency which was a source of great frustration to him.

The early onset of schizophrenia had stymied his development, resulting in underdeveloped social, emotional, vocational, leisure, and independent living skills (i.e., problems with internal capabilities), which rendered him dependent on his parents. Furthermore, the strong cultural identity and connection to the Māori world that he had developed while living with his paternal grandparents, and which supported the adaptive attainment of multiple primary human goods, was disrupted when he returned to the care of his parents. Hemi's removal from the traditional cultural environment in which he was raised, and subsequent feelings of disconnection from his culture (i.e., problems with external capacity), resulted in a loss of identity, belonging, and sense of continuity. While he had flourished under the love, support, and attention of his grandparents, the emotional climate of his new home was distant and hostile (i.e., problems with external capacity).

Collectively, these internal and external obstacles to the attainment of primary goods left many gaps in Hemi's life (i.e., problems with scope) which further undermined his well-being. His passive aggressive behavior toward his mother, through which he sought to assert some control, only fueled the antagonism between them (i.e., problems with means). Hemi's poor compliance with prescribed medications and reluctance to engage with mental health services can also be recognized as attempts to exercise agency.

7.5.3 GLM Approach to Rehabilitation

Hemi came into a new program some 10 years after he was compulsorily detained in a New Zealand forensic hospital. By then he had undergone a range of interventions (e.g., pharmacotherapy, illness education, offense work, stress management training), but his engagement in treatment had been poor and it was doubtful whether he had made any real progress in his rehabilitation. He continued to lack insight into his illness and offending, would periodically secrete his medication, and remained preoccupied with his entrenched delusions. His mental state was highly sensitive to stress, much of which seemed to arise from frustration about being told what to do and the expectation that he would attend therapeutic programs where he saw no purpose. He coped by adopting an outwardly compliant demeanor, while surreptitiously circumventing hospital rules and policies, engaging only superficially with therapeutic interventions, and withholding important information from his treatment team.

There appeared to be little to be gained from keeping Hemi in the hospital, and staff began discussing a plan to transition him back into the community. They were aware that he had several dynamic risk factors that would need to be carefully managed if he was to be safely reintegrated into society. These risk factors were his poor insight, unresponsiveness to treatment, noncompliance with medication, nonengagement with counseling and therapeutic programs, susceptibility to stress, and lack of personal support. Several core issues (i.e., problems with internal and external capacity) appeared to underpin most of these risk factors: his resentment of and subtle opposition to the requests and directions of others (especially authority figures), a perception that therapeutic interventions and medication were of no benefit to him, difficulties identifying and expressing negative emotions, underdeveloped social skills and difficulty developing friendships, and ostracism from his siblings and wider family.

The mapping table (Table 7.1) provides a snapshot of Hemi's life in hospital at the outset of his engagement in GLM work. As can be seen, his overarching primary goods of creativity and community were only partially met in hospital, and other heavily weighted primary goods such as agency were largely absent. What was also apparent, is that Hemi had limited means to satisfy a range of other primary goods, resulting in some problems with scope.

Consistent with his desire to have more control over his life, Hemi identified that he would like to live in his own home when he left hospital. Finding suitable accommodation proved difficult, but his forensic team eventually managed to find him a small apartment within a community-based complex for people with mental health issues that provided on-site staff support. This type of living arrangement satisfied Hemi's need for independence while simultaneously providing him with a sense of community, which he also yearned for. Hemi accepted that taking antipsychotic medication and engaging with forensic and residential staff were prerequisites for living in the community. Despite his ongoing lack of insight into his illness, he was usually compliant with these conditions.

With community housing now secured, Hemi's treatment team then turned their attention to exploring how they could support him to access other prioritized primary goods, especially creativity and community. Conversations with Hemi highlighted a strong desire to reconnect to his Māori culture and an interest in learning the art of *whakairo* (Māori carving). It was subsequently agreed that learning Māori carving should be placed at the center of Hemi's good life plan. Not only would this bring together Hemi's cultural and creative priorities, but it would also provide him with opportunities to satisfy the primary good of community. Attendance at a Māori carving course would introduce Hemi to a group of people with similar interests. Once he developed expertise in his craft, he could potentially become part of a community of Māori artists. Importantly, the practical identities of developing Māori carver and artist would provide him with a narrative that incorporated his core

Table 7.1 Hemi's GLM mapping table

Primary goods	Importance (high, moderate, low)	Means (appropriate & inappropriate)	Internal strengths	Internal obstacles	External strengths	External obstacles	Relationship to offending/mental illness (related, unrelated, protective)
Physical Well-being	Low	Attends exercise group	Desire to increase fitness	Struggles with motivation	Availability of ward exercise program	Restricted range of exercise options	Related
Relationships	Moderate	Interacts with key worker Seeks out fellow client for conversation	Converses about topics that interest him	Struggles to express emotions, poor social skills	Opportunities to develop relationship skills in hospital	Limited opportunities to meet like-minded people; ostracism from family	Related
Community	High	Attends Māori cultural group	Motivated to join groups that cater to his interests	Not confident in groups	Opportunities to engage in cultural activities with others	Lack of opportunities to join groups that cater to his specific interests	Unrelated
Excellence in work	Moderate		Has good work ethic	Very little work experience		Little opportunity to explore work options in hospital	Unrelated
Play	Moderate	Attends art group Enjoys watching TV Draws	Has several interests		Some opportunities for leisure Activities	Restricted range of leisure activities	Unrelated
Creativity	High	Attends art group	Inventive, imaginative, good problem-solver, Practical skills		Some arts and craft groups available in hospital	Lack of opportunity to pursue creative pursuits that interest him most in hospital	Unrelated

Personal choice and independence	High	Engages in decisions about his rehabilitation; Secretes medication; Circumvents rules; Withholds information from staff	Knows what he wants; Needs little direction with self-cares	Struggles with authority figures		Hospital environment curtails agency	Related
Knowledge	Moderate	Learning about Māori culture	Motivation to learn more about culture and interests		Some opportunities to further cultural knowledge	No access to the internet; limited access to books	Unrelated
Peace of mind	Moderate	Engagement in creative pursuits; Withdrawal; Avoidance		Mental illness; Sensitivity to stress; difficulties with emotion regulation			Related
Happiness	Moderate	Art group, Drawing, Watching TV	Engaging in some creative pursuits promotes pleasure			Restricted opportunities for pleasure in hospital	Unrelated
Spirituality	Moderate	Māori cultural group	Knowledge of Māori culture				Unrelated

values and interests, bolster his cultural identity, and provide direction for the development of a prosocial and fulfilling good life plan.

Enrollment in an extended Māori carving course at the local *wananga* (tertiary institution catering for Māori learning needs) would also broaden the scope of Hemi's life by providing access to a range of other primary goods. For example, learning the techniques, history, and *tikanga* (correct procedure) associated with *whakairo* from experienced Māori carvers would enrich his understanding of Māori culture (i.e., primary good of knowledge), provide access to a group of peers and a source of social support (i.e., primary good of relationships), and help him become proficient in his craft over time (i.e., primary goods of mastery and play). Further, the opportunity to work on personal projects later in the course would provide further scope for innovation and experimentation (i.e., primary good of creativity), while allowing him to work more independently (i.e., primary good of agency).

Crucially, attending the Māori carving course required Hemi to work on the core problems underpinning his dynamic risk factors. For example, in order to make progress in his art, he had to learn to accept direction and feedback from his tutors and to ask for help. His personal projects were a vehicle for self-expression and provided a means of talking about himself to others. Encouragement to mix with the other students, combined with some social skills coaching by his tutors, helped him to build his interpersonal skills and social confidence and provided access to social support. Finally, regular check-ins with his tutors and forensic team provided opportunities to discuss stressful aspects of the course and ways of coping that he could later apply.

Despite having spent over a decade in a forensic hospital, Hemi adapted remarkably well to his new lifestyle. On completion of the Māori carving course, he continued to develop his art, setting up a small Internet-based business, and exhibiting his work in local galleries. He maintained contact with one of the tutors from his course, whom he regarded as a mentor, and periodically met with some of the other students.

This case vignette demonstrates how designing an intervention plan around individuals' personal priorities embedded within practical identities can both reduce their risk of recidivism and consolidate new ways of living. It also highlights the synergy between the three aims of the forensic version of the GLM. Promoting Hemi's well-being, by supporting his goals of living in his own home and becoming a Māori carver, supported his recovery from mental illness and consequently helped to reduce his risk of recidivism. Importantly, the decisive rehabilitation work occurred outside the therapy room (and hospital) and was made possible by providing Hemi with the opportunities to enact his version of a good life. This calls into question the notion that therapy-induced change is the critical factor and subsequent reentry into society follows from this. This type of thinking can lead to impasses with individuals like Hemi who fail to engage with standard therapies and programs.

7.6 Conclusions

The GLM offers a promising new paradigm to approach the complexities of forensic practice. It has the potential to overcome the major weaknesses of the traditional approach to forensic care, which have arisen largely due to a lack of available practice frameworks. This theoretical void has meant that, when designing rehabilitation programs, practitioners have tended to select a range of interventions based on FSUs' specific diagnoses and problems (including mental illness and offending behavior), which are derived from antagonistic theoretical orientations. However, this practice is problematic, because it does not provide a theoretically cohesive foundation for rehabilitation planning. Furthermore, it carries the very real risk that forensic rehabilitation will be carried out in an unsystematic, ad hoc, and/or mechanical manner with little reference to the person themselves.

The GLM focuses as much on the person as on their offending and mental illness. The attention to an individual's life values, aspirations, and strengths, alongside their problems is likely to be more appealing to FSUs, bolstering their sense of agency and enhancing their engagement in treatment, motivation to change, and relationships with staff. For practitioners, the GLM offers a comprehensive practice framework that facilitates a cohesive understanding of the person and their core rehabilitation needs and provides guidance on every aspect of forensic practice.

References

Ackerman, S. J., & Hilsenroth, M. J. (2003). A review of therapist characteristics and techniques positively impacting the therapeutic alliance. *Clinical Psychology Review, 23*, 1–33. https://doi.org/10.1016/S0272-7358(02)00146-0

Andrews, D. A., & Bonta, J. (2010). *The psychology of criminal conduct* (5th ed.). LexisNexis.

Andrews, D. A., Bonta, J., & Hoge, R. D. (1990). Classification for effective rehabilitation: Rediscovering psychology. *Criminal Justice and Behavior, 17*, 19–52. https://doi.org/10.1177/0093854890017001004

Barnao, M., Robertson, P., & Ward, T. (2010). Good Lives Model applied to a forensic population. *Psychiatry, Psychology and Law, 17*, 202–217. https://doi.org/10.1080/13218710903421274

Barnao, M., & Ward, T. (2015). Sailing uncharted seas without a compass: A review of interventions in forensic mental health. *Aggression and Violent Behavior, 22*, 77–86. https://doi.org/10.1016/j.avb.2015.04.009

Barnao, M., Ward, T., & Casey, S. (2015). Looking beyond the illness: Forensic service users' perceptions of rehabilitation. *Journal of Interpersonal Violence, 30*, 1025–1045. https://doi.org/10.1177/0886260514539764

Barnao, M., Ward, T., & Casey, S. (2016). Taking the good life to the institution: Forensic service users' perceptions of the Good Lives Model. *International Journal of Offender Therapy and Comparative Criminology, 60*, 766–786. https://doi.org/10.1177/0306624X15570027

Barnao, M., Ward, T., & Robertson, P. (2016). The Good Lives Model: A new paradigm for forensic mental health. *Psychiatry, Psychology and Law, 23*(2), 288–301. https://doi.org/10.1080/13218719.2015.1054923

Bentall, R. P. (2003). *Madness explained*. Penguin Press.

Björkman, T., Hansson, L., Svensson, B., & Berglund, I. (1995). What is important in psychiatric outpatient care? Quality of care from the patient's perspective. *International Journal for Quality in Health Care, 7*, 355–362.
Blackburn, R. (2004). "What works" with mentally disordered offenders. *Psychology, Crime, and Law, 10*, 297–308. https://doi.org/10.1080/10683160410001662780
Bressington, D., Stewart, B., Beer, D., & MacInnes, D. (2011). Levels of service user satisfaction in secure settings: A survey of the association between perceived social climate, perceived therapeutic relationship and satisfaction with forensic services. *International Journal of Nursing Studies, 48*, 1349–1356. https://doi.org/10.1016/j.ijnurstu.2011.05.011
Brooker, C., & Ullmann, B. (2008). *Out of sight, out of mind. The state of mental healthcare in prison*. Policy Exchange.
Büsselmann, M., Nigel, S., Otte, S., Lutz, M., Franke, I., Dudeck, M., et al. (2020). High quality of life reduces depression, hopelessness, and suicide ideations in patients in forensic psychiatry. *Frontiers in Psychiatry, 10*, 1014. https://doi.org/10.3389/fpsyt.2019.01014
Byrne, G. (2020). How the Good Lives Model can complement mentalization-based treatments for individuals who have offended with anti-social personality disorder and general forensic mental health needs: Practice update. *International Journal of Offender Therapy and Comparative Criminology, 64*(15), 1587. https://doi.org/10.1177/0306624X209280
Chow, W. S., & Priebe, S. (2013). Understanding psychiatric institutionalization: A conceptual review. *BMC Psychiatry, 13*(1), 169. https://doi.org/10.1186/1471-244X-13-169
Clark, D. A. (2000). *Theory manual for enhanced thinking skills: Prepared for the joint prison accreditation panel*. Home Office.
Corrigan, P. W. (2004). Target-specific stigma change; a strategy for impacting mental illness stigma. *Psychiatric Rehabilitation Journal, 28*, 113–121.
De Smet, S., Van Hecke, N., Verte, D., Broekaert, E., Ryan, D., & Vandevelde, S. (2015). Treatment and control: A qualitative study of older mentally ill offenders' perceptions on their detention and care trajectory. *International Journal of Offender Therapy and Comparative Criminology, 59*, 964–985. https://doi.org/10.1177/0306624X14521129
Emmons, R. A. (1999). *The psychology of ultimate concerns*. Guilford Press.
Farnworth, L., Nikitin, L., & Fossey, E. (2004). Being in a secure forensic psychiatric unit: Every day is the same, killing time or making the most of it. *British Journal of Occupational Therapy, 67*, 430–438. https://doi.org/10.1177/030802260406701003
Fioravanti, M., Bianchi, V., & Cinti, M. E. (2012). Cognitive deficits in schizophrenia: An updated meta-analysis of the scientific evidence. *BMC Psychiatry, 12*, 64. https://doi.org/10.1186/1471-244X-12-64
Franke, I., Büsselmann, M., Streb, J., & Dudeck, M. (2019). Perceived institutional restrain is associated with psychological distress in forensic psychiatric inpatients. *Frontiers in Psychiatry, 10*, 410. https://doi.org/10.3389/fpsyt.2019.00410
Gannon, T. A., King, T., Miles, H., Lockerbie, L., & Willis, G. M. (2011). Good Lives sexual offender treatment for mentally disordered offenders. *The British Journal of Forensic Practice, 13*, 153–166. https://doi.org/10.1108/14636641111157805
Hare Duke, L., Furtado, V., Guo, B., & Völlm, B. A. (2018). Long-stay in forensic-psychiatric care in the UK. *Social Psychiatry and Psychiatric Epidemiology, 53*(3), 313–321. https://doi.org/10.1007/s00127-017-1473-y
Hart, S., Sturmey, P., Logan, C., & McMurran, M. (2011). Forensic case formulation. *International Journal of Forensic Mental Health, 10*, 118–126. https://doi.org/10.1080/14999013.2011.577137
Hodge, J. E., & Renswick, S. J. (2002). Motivating mentally disordered offenders. In M. McMurran (Ed.), *Motivating offenders to change: A guide to enhancing engagement in therapy* (pp. 221–234). John Wiley & Sons Ltd.
Hodgins, S. (2002). Research priorities in forensic mental health. *International Journal of Forensic Mental Health, 1*, 7–23. https://doi.org/10.1080/14999013.2002.10471157

Hörberg, U., Sjogren, R., & Dahlberg, K. (2012). To be strategically struggling against resignation: The lived experience of being cared for in forensic psychiatric care. *Issues in Mental Health Nursing, 33*, 743–751. https://doi.org/10.3109/01612840.2012.704623

Jacobson, N., & Greenley, D. (2001). What is recovery? A conceptual model and explication. *Psychiatric Services, 52*, 482–485.

Johansson, H., & Eklund, M. (2003). Patients' opinion on what constitutes good psychiatric care. *Scandinavian Journal of Caring Sciences, 17*, 339–346.

Layard, R., Chisholm, D., Patel, V., & Saxena, S. (2013). Mental illness and unhappiness. In J. Helliwell, R. Layard, & J. Sachs (Eds.), *World happiness report 2013*. Earth Institute, Columbia University. Retrieved from: http://ssrn.com/abstract=2336397

Leach, M. J. (2005). Rapport: A key to treatment success. *Complementary Therapies in Clinical Practice, 11*, 262–265. https://doi.org/10.1016/j.ctcp.2005.05.005

Leaming, N., & Willis, G. M. (2016). The Good Lives Model: New avenues for Māori rehabilitation? *Sexual Abuse in Australia and New Zealand, 7*(1), 59–69.

Lilja, L., & Hellzen, O. (2008). Former patients' experience of psychiatric care: A qualitative investigation. *International Journal of Mental Health Nursing, 17*, 279–286. https://doi.org/10.1111/j.1447-0349.2008.00544.x

Lutz, M., Zani, D., Fritz, M., Dudeck, M., & Franke, I. (2022). A review and comparative analysis of the risk-needs-responsivity, good lives, and recovery models in forensic psychiatric treatment. *Frontiers in Psychiatry, 13*, 988905. https://doi.org/10.3389/fpsyt.2022.988905

McKenna, B. (2020). Cultural safety: There is no turning back! *Journal of Psychiatric and Mental Health Nursing, 27*(5), 495–496.

Palijan, T. Z., Radeljak, S., Kovac, M., & Kovacevic, D. (2010). Relationship between comorbidity and violence risk assessment in forensic psychiatry—The implication of neuroimaging studies. *Psychiatria Danubina, 22*, 253–256.

Pouncey, C. L., & Lukens, J. M. (2010). Madness versus badness: The ethical tension between the recovery movement and forensic psychiatry. *Theoretical Medicine and Bioethics, 31*, 93–105.

Rice, M., & Harris, G. (1997). The treatment of mentally disordered offenders. *Psychology, Public Policy, and Law, 3*, 126–183. https://doi.org/10.1037/1076-8971.3.1.126

Robertson, P., Barnao, M., & Ward, T. (2011). Rehabilitation frameworks in forensic mental health. *Aggression and Violent Behavior, 16*, 472–484. https://doi.org/10.1016/j.avb.2011.03.003

Ross, R. R., & Fabiano, E. A. (1985). *Time to think: A cognitive model of delinquency prevention and offender rehabilitation*. Institute of Social science and Arts.

Rutherford, M., & Duggan, S. (2008). Forensic mental health services: Facts and figures on current provision. *The British Journal of Forensic Practice, 10*, 4–10. https://doi.org/10.1108/14636646200800020

Simons, D.A., McCullar, B., & Tyler, C. (2006, September). Evaluation of the Good Lives Model approach to treatment planning. Paper presented at the *25th Annual Association for the Treatment of Sexual Abusers Research and Treatment Conference*, Chicago.

Simpson, A. I. F., & Penney, S. R. (2018). Recovery and forensic care: Recent advances and future directions. *Criminal Behavior and Mental Health, 28*(5), 383. https://doi.org/10.1002/cbm.2090

Spitzer, C., Chevalier, C., Gillner, M., Freyberger, H., & Barnow, S. (2006). Complex posttraumatic stress disorder and child maltreatment in forensic inpatients. *Forensic Psychiatry & Psychology, 17*, 204–216. https://doi.org/10.1080/14789940500497743

Strauss-Hughes, A., Ward, T., & Neha, T. (2022). Considering practice frameworks for culturally diverse populations in the correctional domain. *Aggression and Violent Behavior, 63*, 101673. https://doi.org/10.1016/j.avb.2021.101673

Ward, T. (2013). Addressing the dual relationship problem in forensic and correctional practice. *Aggression and Violent Behavior, 18*, 92–100. https://doi.org/10.1016/j.avb.2012.10.006

Ward, T., & Durrant, R. (2021). Practice frameworks in correctional psychology: Translating causal theories and normative assumptions into practice. *Aggression and Violent Behavior, 58*, 101612. https://doi.org/10.1016/j.avb.2021.101612

Ward, T., & Maruna, S. (2007). *Rehabilitation: Beyond the risk paradigm*. Routledge.
Ward, T., & Stewart, C. A. (2003). The treatment of sex offenders: Risk management and good lives. *Professional Psychology: Research and Practice, 34*, 353–360.
Ward, T., & Syversen, K. (2009). Human dignity and vulnerable agency: An ethical framework for forensic practice. *Aggression and Violent Behavior, 14*, 94–105. https://doi.org/10.1016/j.avb.2008.12.002
Ward, T., Mann, R. E., & Gannon, T. A. (2007). The good lives model of offender rehabilitation: Clinical implications. *Aggression and Violent Behavior, 12*, 87–107.
World Health Organization. (2013). *Mental health action plan 2013–2020*. WHO. Document Production Services. Retrieved from: http://www.who.int/iris/bitstream/10665/89966/1/9789241506021_eng

Chapter 8
Case Examples

8.1 Introduction

This chapter reviews applications of the good lives model (GLM) with clients. Based on the authors' common experiences, these cases are fictitious and describe individuals, and then explore the primary human goods (PHGs) important to them and that were implicated in their abusive behaviors. Next is an exploration of the strengths and obstacles that clients experienced on the way to achieving their vision of a good life. Finally, ideas for GLM-based treatment are proposed. Some of the tools described in Chap. 3 are applied in practice.

8.2 Tommy

8.2.1 Introduction

Tommy is 21 years old. He resides with his mother and younger brother (13 years old) in a medium-sized European city. He has received a preliminary conviction (explained below) for distributing nude images of his ex-girlfriend, Anja. They had been together for about 1 year. Tommy distributed these images through social media that he knew both of their friends would see. Upon discovery, he told authorities that he wanted to get back at her for dumping him, and secretly hoped that it might lead her to contact him to resolve their differences and repair their relationship. He has no previous criminal history.

Tommy recently entered into another sexual relationship with a same-aged woman, Bella, prior to his arrest. Although she has not left him because of his crime, their relationship is at a standstill. Also noteworthy is that after he was arrested and

T. Ward et al., *The Good Lives Model of Correctional Rehabilitation*,
Advances in Preventing and Treating Violence and Aggression,
https://doi.org/10.1007/978-3-031-95559-4_8

was awaiting his sentence, Tommy made a violent suicide attempt. He took an overdose of medication and stabbed himself with a knife. He stated at the time that his life had become impossible to manage and that suicide was the only means he had for taking control of it. He also hoped that others would miss him and view him favorably.

Tommy presented himself for treatment in a confused state, saying, on the one hand, that he regretted that his act of revenge had made others unhappy, and on the other hand that it was the only course of action available to him and that he would consider doing it again if the same circumstances recurred. Although Tommy received a preliminary conviction, he could avoid a full conviction (one that would be part of his permanent criminal record) by participating in treatment.

8.2.2 Background Information

Tommy grew up in a family that faced poverty and its effects every day. Although he has no known history of sexual victimization, his family life was tumultuous. In his earliest years, he witnessed his parents arguing and sometimes physically fighting. His mother started to develop medical conditions that would progress in severity through Tommy's childhood, which made the family's financial and emotional situation even more bleak. It is entirely possible that Tommy witnessed his father sexually assaulting his mother, but this is uncertain because Tommy's memory is vague.

Tommy was 8 years old when his younger brother, Francis, was born. Although welcome in the family, the newborn Francis presented new responsibilities and obligations at the very time that their mother's health was deteriorating. Tommy's father became even more stressed and left the family shortly thereafter. They never heard from him again. His departure and absence were felt every day afterwards; however, the others rarely spoke of this because of the more immediate threats that they faced.

Not surprisingly, Tommy's performance in school suffered. He was diagnosed with attention deficit hyperactivity disorder (ADHD) by the time he was 10 years old. His teachers were patient with him and supported him to the best of their abilities. He was eventually able to graduate high school but entered the work force instead of pursuing further education.

Tommy's daily life from the ages of eight until 18 was marked by doing his best to take care of his mother and to help his brother. This meant that he was constantly on the go, taking care of others as their immediate needs arose and only rarely experiencing a sense of calm, inner peace, fun, or other states of happiness and pleasure. Interestingly, Tommy developed many skills at the expense of others. His efforts to live and survive each day provided him with a strong work ethic that would serve him well in later years. However, his focus on problem-solving in the present moment left him with almost no skills for scheduling, planning, or anticipating problems that might arise. His remarkable resilience at getting through each day also meant that he had few resources for regulating his emotions, for example, being able to calm himself down. In many ways, his life was like running a marathon every day without adequate rest or strategies for pacing himself.

Looking back in treatment years later, Tommy has come to understand that he had never known how anxious he was or how little rest he had gotten. It is no wonder that the school had diagnosed him with attention deficit hyperactivity disorder and that his efforts to manage family adversity and precocious responsibilities had resulted in poor school performance and difficulties structuring his life. Sadly, his hard work has been offset by his missing appointments and issues with concentration, with the result that he is seen as unreliable by his family and girlfriends.

When Tommy finished high school, at the age of 18, he went to work at a restaurant along a highway. He has held this position for over 3 years, including since his arrest. The nature of his work is difficult: Tommy works with day contracts, which means he does not know his working hours for the next day until the evening before. He focusses very hard on this job and aims to do it well. He strives to become the manager of this highway restaurant, so he does everything that he is asked for.

Tommy met Anja when he was 19 years old. At first, she was a welcome respite from a life filled with work, taking care of his family, and attempting to establish himself firmly in the workplace. He particularly appreciated that in addition to having someone to confide in, he felt calm and safe in her presence. Their relationship provided a sense of inner peace as well as states of happiness and pleasure that had long been virtually unknown to him.

At the start of their relationship, Tommy convinced Anja to pose nude for several photographs. He also recorded them having sex on his phone. At the time, Anja had hoped that doing this would help ensure a deeper relationship. Over time, she became uncertain that this had been a good idea. She asked him to show her that he had deleted all the photos and videos. At first, he declined. Later, he claimed unconvincingly that he had done this, leaving her wondering whether she could trust him.

As much as Tommy had come to depend on Anja for emotional support (as well as happiness and pleasure), he did not notice the subtle signs that she was increasingly unhappy with their relationship. From Anja's perspective, Tommy's difficulties with planning and problem-solving skills, combined with few opportunities for employment that would ensure a more stable and predictable lifestyle, were concerning. His apparent deception around deleting the photos led Anja to end the relationship.

Tommy's reaction to Anja's leaving the relationship caused him anguish and anxiety. He quickly became filled with rage, a sense of grievance, and thoughts of revenge. It did not take long for him to decide that sending the nude photos of Anja (which he had stored on an external hard drive) would be a good way to get back at her. Underneath his momentary rage and grief, Tommy came to believe that he was unlovable and unworthy, and that the world around him was not to be trusted. Against that backdrop, distributing Anja's photos made sense to him. It seemed that this was the sole action he could take that would demonstrate a sense of agency and self-efficacy.

It did not take long for Anja to call the police and for Tommy to be arrested. He was briefly processed by the police and allowed to return home prior to a court hearing. Upon arriving home, Tommy attempted suicide. After swallowing an overdose of medicine, he stabbed himself. His neighbors heard him scream and attempted to check in on him. When they received no response, they called the police and Tommy was hospitalized.

8.2.3 Assessment

After receiving a preliminary conviction, which would not go on his criminal record if he completed treatment, Tommy was referred for an assessment to determine his risks and treatment needs. It was understood that Tommy's crime appeared more motivated by revenge than by intrinsic sexual gratification, thus, the referral questions were related to what kinds of risks Tommy posed, how best to understand him, and how best to provide treatment. The initial risk evaluation used the Level of Service/Case Management Inventory (as a measure of risk for general criminality; Andrews et al., n.d.) and Sexual Violence Risk—20, Version 2 (to assess risk of sexual re-offense; Hart & Boer, 2021). This assessment of static and dynamic factors took place during the judicial process.

Initial results placed Tommy in the low–moderate risk range. Static factors examined included his age (21) and the fact that he hadn't lived with a lover in a marital-type relationship for 2 years. An assessment of dynamic factors highlighted areas such as Tommy's intimate relationship history, significant social influences, negative emotionality, and problem-solving skills. His recent loss of a social support (his prior girlfriend) and rapidly escalating negative affect (resulting in a suicide attempt) were also noted.

The evaluation next examined Tommy's strengths, positive attributes, and protective factors against further crimes of a sexual nature. The evaluator used the SAPROF-SO (Kelley et al., 2022). This measure identified the following protective factors that could mitigate risk and assist Tommy in both his treatment and his life generally:

- Positive attitudes toward rules and regulations (apart from his crime)
- Good sexual self-regulation
- Prosocial sexual interests
- A prosocial sexual identity
- Some capacity for relationships
- A history of goal-directed living (his crime notwithstanding)
- A work history
- Strong motivation to improve his life and manage risks

At this point of the assessment, Tommy was found to have a low–moderate baseline of risk, with some likely mitigation by his protective factors. The available risk assessment measures only tell part of the story needed for careful, effortful assessment and intervention, as will be discussed below.

8.2.4 GLM-Specific Assessment

The evaluator (E) continued to interview Tommy (T) in accordance with the GLM assessment interview and mapping tool described in Chap. 3. As a sample:

(E) Who do you most want to spend time with?

(T) Right now, Bella is my primary focus. I need to show her that I can make my life work and our relationship work. She's told me that she is willing to wait for all this legal activity to settle down, but she's obviously not going to wait forever. At the same time, I really want things to be right between me, my brother, and my mother. I really want a second chance there.

(E) It's not just that you want better relationships, you also want to make right any past wrongs you've caused.

(T) Yeah. And I want to communicate better with the people I work with, of course. I try hard, but I'm not always good at that.

(E) What's gotten in the way of your relationships in the past?

(T) What hasn't? With my family I was always trying hard to keep money coming in. I mean, I never really got to talk about how my father just left us. I am determined never to do that to anyone important to me. But I've just never had the time because my day contract work means I constantly have to do what I can when it's available. But then there's the fact that I always just seem not to notice when the time is right to be with others. Anja and I mostly just connected around sex. I try to hide it, but I'm just not that good at talking with people (looking down, sadly).

(E) What would need to happen for you to talk with people and form deeper connections?

(T) I guess the first thing would be to structure my time better. No one believes they can rely on me, and they're not wrong. If I were better organized, that would be a good start. Honestly, the rest—I think—is mostly about practicing, like learning how to manage a restaurant, it's all in the practice, learning the skills.

(E) Here in the program, we have a class on organizational skills, things for managing daily life. In treatment, we also have a focus on practicing relationship skills. Would either of those work for you?

(T) At this point, I'm really willing to try anything. Especially if it will help me in front of that judge! (smiles).

(E) That sounds great; I can make sure that happens. Just a couple more questions?

(T) Okay.

(E) How will you know that things are getting better?

(T) I will check in with Bella and she will tell me that she's happy with my progress.

(E) And how will others know that things are getting better? What will they notice?

(T) They'll feel like they can trust me.

The evaluator continued exploring all of the PHGs in turn. Tommy then further explored his life history, and the offense process itself. At first, Tommy and the evaluator discussed how his experiences have combined into vulnerabilities that:

- Could make further offending more likely to occur in unfavorable conditions
- Function as barriers to achieving good life goals

These vulnerabilities included:

- His problematic relationship with, and subsequent absence of, his father, which has remained unresolved for him

- A history of having a chaotic family environment, including possible exposure to abuse
- The lack of emotional support from his family
- A lack of more advanced employment opportunities
- A very stressful current job
- Few coping skills
- Financial pressures

Challenges in Tommy's early life development limited his capacity for secure attachments with others in his life. These same events appear to have left him with the implicit theory that the world can be dangerous and out of control and that others are not to be trusted. He has had difficulty negotiating relationships with women, specifically trusting and being trusted by them.

Tommy clearly needs help managing relationships with others, including people he interacts with in the community and those close to him. The broader goal became helping Tommy to experience himself as competent within his personal relationships and to relate to others empathically. Attaining skills in this area would significantly reduce his risk.

Tommy's other risk/need domain involves his ability to balance his relationships with others with his own experience of independence, mastery (excellence in work; excellence at play), and living and surviving. As Tommy and his treatment team (including the evaluator and his therapist) would come to understand him:

- At the time of life when others form secure attachments with caregivers, Tommy was experiencing a chaotic family environment.
- When others were forming friendships in school, Tommy was learning that those close to him either left him or were emotionally unavailable.
- At an age when others were learning to read and write, Tommy's family was impoverished, his mother ill, his father leaving, and his brother entering the world and needing care.
- At the time of his development, where others were learning relationship and courtship skills such as socializing in groups and dating, Tommy was experiencing social and emotional isolation.
- At those ages when other adolescents were developing independent living skills, Tommy had to focus on helping his family to survive.
- At a time when others had built the resilience to cope with relationship problems and failures, Tommy was still living in the mindset of self-protection.

8.2.5 Primary Human Goods

Given the information learned so far, Tommy's most prioritized PHGs prior to his arrest were:

- Living and surviving (evident in his upbringing, surviving a chaotic home life, and desperately seeking to provide for his family)
- Being good at work (to this point in his life, this is primarily connected to the other PHGs of living and surviving and excellence in agency)
- Relatedness (evident in his attempts to form and maintain relationships)

Tommy focused less on:

- Excellence in agency (autonomy; evident in his taking charge over situations, including in his relationship with Anja)
- Inner peace (evident in his cannabis use)
- States of happiness and pleasure

PHGs that Tommy had not prioritized (primarily because he was so focused on his most prioritized PHGs) were:

- Knowledge
- Creativity
- Being good at play
- Community
- Spirituality

Across his life, Tommy's pursuit of the PHGs showed that the coherence of his implicit good life plan (GLP) was almost entirely vertical. As a result of surviving a chaotic and broken home, facing financial hardships, and challenges in his relationships with others, he prioritized a narrow range of PHGs well above others. Whether these were PHGs that he would have prioritized had he grown up under less severe circumstances is a question he could eventually explore in therapy. One cost of these circumstances was that Tommy was never able to develop horizontal coherence in his GLP. In other words, there has not been explicit, consistent relationships between his PHGs. For example, Tommy's pursuit of living and surviving and being good at work frequently clashed with his relationships. As noted in Chap. 1, a life that has low coherence is likely to lead to frustration and harm to the individual concerned. This may also lead to a life lacking in overall sense of purpose and meaning, as is exactly the case with Tommy.

Tommy's life is striking for its lack of secondary goods to achieve the PHGs. An initial accounting is:

PHG of living and surviving. Tommy's secondary goods include:

- Working to earn money
- Developing skills across his life to identify threats to his well-being in his environment (at the cost of developing skills for anticipating and solving problems and planning for the future)

PHG of being good at work. Tommy's secondary goods include:

- Upskilling and finding better employment (to date, he has not been successful with this)

PHG of relatedness. Tommy's secondary goods include:

- Sexual behavior (including photographing Anja)
- Efforts to provide for his family
- Attempts to get along with co-workers

PHG of inner peace. Tommy's secondary goods include:

- Sex
- Cannabis

PHG of states of happiness and pleasure. Tommy's secondary goods include:

- Sex
- Cannabis

PHG of knowledge. Tommy shows little need for knowledge. However, he does show that he would like to talk more about the past, e.g., when father left, to gain a better understanding of it.

PHG of creativity. Tommy reports that he has virtually no secondary goods related to this, with the possible exceptions of occasional sexual novelty.

PHG of being good at play. Tommy reports almost no secondary good besides checking the help-wanted advertisements.

PHG of Community. Tommy has felt nearly completely cut off from his community except for occasional interactions with his neighbors.

PHG of spirituality. Tommy has not been able to identify secondary goods and feels that his only purpose in life so far has been to provide for his family and 1 day become married and have children.

As the assessment process continued, Tommy and the evaluator explored the PHGs implicated in Tommy's offense. These were:

- Relatedness (evident in his attempts to re-connect with his ex-girlfriend). The associated secondary good is the use of inappropriate/harmful means to control Anja through releasing nude photos of her.
- Excellence in agency (evident in his attempts to control the relationship and its break-up). The associated secondary good manifests through inappropriate/ harmful means of seeking revenge by releasing Anja's nude photos.

8.2.6 *Obstacles to the Primary Human Goods Involved in Tommy's Offense*

Tommy and the evaluator discussed how the challenges of his early life and more recent circumstances had combined to help explain his harmful and illegal behaviors. First, Tommy had experienced both internal lack of capacity and external lack of capacity. His life circumstances had prevented him from achieving many developmental tasks and acquiring the skills to lead a good life. As a result of lacking capacity, Tommy developed a narrow scope to his good life, evident in the PHGs that he did not seek to achieve as actively as he did others. Without a focus on the PHGs of excellence at play, knowledge, community, creativity, and spirituality, Tommy became at increasingly high risk not only for problematic and harmful behaviors but for not living up to his full potential as a person.

The subsequent lack of vertical and horizontal coherence resulted in conflicts between his goals and the means he used to attain them. He was unable to balance excellence in agency with relatedness with the result that the means he used to attain one would conflict with another goal. For example, pursuing agency by causing further harm to his relationship with Anja in revenge for her leaving him, all the while lacking the skills to attempt reconciliation, resulted in a crisis of agency in which he felt he could not continue on his own.

In the end, Tommy used completely inappropriate means to achieve PHGs that are common to all human beings. This use of inappropriate means had the ironic effect of harming Tommy, his family, and Anja. His subsequent legal status has further impeded his relationship with Bella.

A closer look at these obstacles was helpful in laying the foundation for treatment planning:

- *Lack of internal and external capacity*: Tommy had few opportunities across his life to develop skills for achieving his good life goals, including inner peace, relatedness, excellence in agency, knowledge, happiness, excellence at work, and excellence at play. His home and school environments offered few opportunities to develop skills in these areas. Having ADHD was a major obstacle in this way. Indeed, it is ironic that Tommy worked so hard to care for a family that was unable to care for him. It is little wonder that he took to cannabis use as his sole means of inner peace outside of his relationship with his girlfriend.
- *Narrow scope*: The resulting lack of skills in turn led to Tommy having a narrow scope through much of his life. He was almost exclusively focused on the goods of living and surviving, excellence in agency, and relatedness. He had little time for anything else. This meant that his efforts at attaining and achieving other goods fell by the wayside.
- *Use of problematic means*: Lacking internal and external capacity to attain goods and with a narrow scope to his good life plan, it would seem to Tommy that he had few options available for feeling in control of his circumstances and for having any chance at convincing Anja to return. Angry and confused, the humiliation of sharing nude images may have seemed like one of the only options he had available. On the one hand, he likely knew it was an extreme option, one that he could never walk away from. On the other hand, it might seem to make sense at the moment.
- *Conflict between goods*: As a result of the above obstacles in combination, Tommy pursued a course of action that, ironically, resulted in severely limiting his own sense of agency and ending that he sought.

Tommy's practical identity (see Chap. 1) revolved around his most highly prized PHGs of relatedness and mastery at work. He considered himself a true family man who works hard and takes good care of his family. He saw himself as a truly dedicated worker who has ideas on how to further grow the company. During the period of time around his offending, each of these seemed harder to achieve. As a result, his life appeared increasingly empty of meaning and purpose.

8.2.7 Good Lives Model Mapping Tool

As the team carried out a joint assessment, they used the collected information to collectively fill out the GLM mapping tool (see Chap. 3). The diverse views of different staff members contribute to a more complete overview (Table 8.1):

The team members developed an overview with its (preliminary) synthesis to create a case formulation (see Chap. 3). They used a narrative form to describe connections between the PHGs, secondary goods, offending behavior, and contexts. This case formulation is part of a collaborative process in which the team and client (see Chap. 6) together prepare a GLM intervention. As the mapping table shows, an investment in internal and external strengths is needed.

8.2.8 GLM Intervention

The judge had given Tommy an opportunity to prevent a full conviction. If he completed a 1-year course of therapy in an outpatient service, he would not be convicted to a sentence of 2 years in prison. He arrived at the therapy center under this obligation.

The staff members had all been trained not just in the practical aspects of applying the GLM but in its theoretical and foundational aspects in order to help them maintain the necessary mindset. To that end, they were aware of areas such as the agent–action–context schema and the six practice commitments described in Chap. 1. They had learned to think of the GLM as a flexible practice framework and not simply a list of principles and protocols. They understood the broader GLM as involving five phases (as described in Chap. 1), many of which might be revisited as treatment progressed, even as the program's focus was on assessment, understanding Tommy's GLP at the time of his offending, developing an intervention plan, and providing therapy.

During the first days, the treatment team reviewed the assessment information to ensure that everyone, especially Tommy, understood the relationship between the offense, the PHGs, the obstacles to achieving the goods, and his strengths and other areas of resiliency. This review process was adapted to Tommy's learning style and other characteristics, including his ADHD. However, it became clear that some

Table 8.1 Tommy's mapping table

Primary goods	Importance	Means	Internal strengths	Internal obstacles	External strengths	External obstacles	Relationship to offending
Life	High	Working to earn money Developing skills to identify threats to his Well-being in his environment	Prosocial sexual identity Surviving skills ("here and now" solutions)	Limited skills for planning and problem-solving Desperate to provide for his family ADHD has prevented developing life skills	There are resources in Tommy's community that he can turn to for help	Poverty Mother's illness Father's absence History of violence in his family, including possible exposure to abuse	Unrelated
Relatedness	High	Sexual behavior (including offense: Controlling Anja by releasing photos) Efforts to provide for his family Relationship with Bella Relationships with colleagues Suicide attempt	Sexual self-regulation Prosocial sexual interests Some capacity for relationships Regrets his act and the damage	Belief that he is unlovable and unworthy Belief that the world around him is not to be trusted Limited capacity for having secure attachments (cf. intimate relationship history) Lack of communication skills ADHD has often interfered with communications and relationships with others	Bella, who he is able to trust Mother and brother are in his life	Problematic relationship with, and absence of father Lack of emotional support from his family Relationship problems with Bella	Related

(continued)

Table 8.1 (continued)

Primary goods	Importance	Means	Internal strengths	Internal obstacles	External strengths	External obstacles	Relationship to offending
Community	Low	He feels nearly completely cut off from his community I'm not sure that this is a secondary good?	Positive attitudes toward rules and regulations (apart from his crime)	Limited skills for planning and problem solving Lack of communication skills Belief that the world around him is not to be trusted	Occasional interactions with his (supportive) neighbors	Few opportunities to develop skills for achieving his good life goals	Unrelated
Excellence/ mastery in work	High	Upskilling and finding better employment (not successful yet)	Skills in problem-solving here and now, and in taking care for others A strong work ethic and persistence A work history	ADHD: Being easily distracted and difficulty making plans Lack of communication skills	With additional training, there are jobs that would be available to Tommy	Lack of more advanced employment opportunities A very stressful current job	Unrelated
Excellence/ mastery in play	Low	Almost no secondary goods besides checking the help-wanted advertisements Is this really play?	Interested in cooking and playing guitar Handling social media	ADHD has interfered with developing areas of interest and continuing with them	There are resources available to Tommy, both online and in his community.	Few opportunities to develop skills for achieving his good life goals	Unrelated
Creativity	Low	Almost no secondary goods besides the possible exceptions of occasional sexual novelty	Interested in cooking and playing guitar Handling social media	Tommy has focused so much on his momentary immediate needs that he has had few opportunities to excel in this area	There are resources available online and in the community that will help Tommy with his creative endeavors	Few opportunities to develop skills for achieving his good life goals, e.g., unpredictable work hours make it difficult to engage in leisure activities	Unrelated

Agency	Moderate	Attempts to control the relationship and its break-up (through releasing Anja's nude photos) Suicide attempt Working hard (to earn money)	Positive attitudes toward rules and regulations (apart from his crime) A history of goal-directed living Strong motivation to improve his life and manage risks	Limited skills for planning and problem-solving ADHD has sometimes interfered with his ability to focus on skills for independent living.	There are treatment programs and social service agencies that can help Tommy develop skills for agency.	Few options available for feeling in control of his circumstances: Mothers' illness and the need for care Financial pressures Depending on a stressful job	Related
Knowledge	Low	Almost no secondary goods besides (wanting) to talk about the past to know more about it	Motivation for a better understanding of his past High school graduation	ADHD has made educational efforts very difficult	Supportive teachers	Few opportunities to develop skills for achieving his good life goals	Unrelated
Inner peace	Moderate	Sex Relationship with Bella Cannabis use Suicide attempt	Motivation to get it right with mother, brother and Bella	Few coping skills to deal with anxiety and negative emotions Longstanding internal effects of history of violence in family ADHD has often interfered with keeping calm	Bella who makes him feel calm	Mothers' illness and the need of care Depending on a stressful job Poverty Few opportunities to develop skills for achieving his good life goals	Unrelated
States of happiness and pleasure	Moderate	Sex Cannabis use Relationship with Bella		Feelings of anxiety and negative emotions Longstanding internal effects of history of violence in family	Bella who makes him feel happy	Mother's illness and the need of care Few opportunities to develop skills for achieving his good life goals	Unrelated

(continued)

Table 8.1 (continued)

Primary goods	Importance	Means	Internal strengths	Internal obstacles	External strengths	External obstacles	Relationship to offending
Spirituality	Low	He feels that his only purpose in life so far has been to provide for his family and 1 day become married and have children	Strong motivation to improve his life and manage risks: He wants to build a meaningful life with Bella, mother, brother, and others.	ADHD has impeded his ability to focus on this area in depth	Resources exist within the community	Some spirituals-inclined resources in the community might be wary of his presence because of his history.	Unrelated

preparatory work needed to take place before beginning to implement a GLM intervention plan.

At first, it was hard for Tommy to concentrate or show up for his appointments on time. His multidisciplinary team tried to use sessions of less than 1 h, structured in advance, in order to ensure his responsiveness to the therapeutic services available to him. The first step was to work on having him become involved in therapy and committed to change. To this end, Tommy and his therapists agreed on using a digital calendar. It turned out that before that, he had never used a calendar at all.

Why a calendar as a first step in the GLP? It allowed him to gain more control over his own life (agency). Everything for Tommy started with something very concrete and specific, such as the difficulty of getting to appointments. He considered these concrete steps possible to realize; he stated he was motivated to try a digital calendar because it could solve some of the problems of being perceived as unreliable by his employer and other important people in his life.

The first course of action was taken. After he began using his calendar for therapy, he started keeping track of his work hours as well. He became more reliable with important others in his life. Being able to keep appointments meant that he became less agitated when they took place. He became better able to invest in relationships with those close to him and found himself in a position to make fewer excuses for any shortcomings.

The multidisciplinary team focused on the calendar to help Tommy gain more control over life. Tommy would use role plays in therapy sessions to practice conversations with his boss. For example, he would receive the message, "Tommy, tomorrow at 6 pm!" Tommy would reply: "I have to see if it fits into my calendar; I will follow up with you shortly." This had the immediate impact of providing him with more structure and more regular sleep, which was important in managing his ADHD and alleviating stress.

As Tommy became settled into the program, his treatment team worked with him to assemble a GLM Intervention plan, which follows below (Table 8.2):

Tommy's good life intervention plan was formed out of a multidisciplinary team discussion with Tommy based on the assessment results and adjusted through the discussions. Instead of completing the assessment and then moving directly to developing and implementing a good life intervention plan, the team first focused on the basics of developing preliminary daily-life skills (such as using the calendar) and on therapeutic engagement due to the short time of Tommy's legal obligation; it was clear that a greater investment in the therapeutic relationship and attention to life skills at the start would make the rest of the good life plan easier to implement.

The resulting sense of agency and relatedness was a start in addressing and reducing the effects of dynamic risk factors (DRF)/criminogenic needs.[1] He could enjoy better relationships with his mother, brother, and girlfriend. This brought about more emotional support and reciprocity in these relationships. He quit his

[1] DRF are signalling devices that indicate problems in achieving important goals, or in GLM language, PHG. They should be viewed as factors that signal problems in motivational systems NOT as causal factors (see Chap. 2).

Table 8.2 Tommy's GLM intervention plan

Primary Goods *Indicate priorities	Interventions		
	Short term: 3 months	Medium term: 6 months	Long term: 1 year or more
Life **	Develop skills for planning and problem-solving. Develop plan for physical exercise according to a schedule. Provide education on nutrition and other daily-life skills	Assist in identifying employment opportunities and housing prospects. Use therapy sessions to discuss how Tommy is using his for planning and problem-solving skills. Review progress on exercise schedule and daily-life skills, making adjustments as needed	Review progress in managing skills acquired and rehearsed over the past year. Ensure that Tommy is managing his employment and housing to the best of his abilities
Agency **	Acquire and rehearse skills for problem-solving, planning for the immediate and long-term future, and flexible thinking skills Develop skills for daily life, including the use of a digital calendar, food preparation, financial management, shopping, and home maintenance	Use therapy to discuss how Tommy is applying the skills he has learned on a weekly basis. Can use role play to explore what does and doesn't work for Tommy Use therapy to review progress and discuss what is and isn't working in daily-life skills. Use therapeutic exercises that bolster these skills. Review progress with case managers who may be able to help identify resources.	As with other PHGs, Tommy can review progress and what Tommy has learned to continue developing his capacities in this area. He can reach work stability, and so more structural, financial stability to manage his life. As with other goals, Tommy and his team can celebrate progress as it occurs
Relatedness **	Participation in relationship skills curricula and education. Focus on skills related to close friends, family, and partners as well as acquaintances	Use therapy sessions to practice and review how Tommy uses skills on a daily basis, in the here and now. Use role play to practice skills as needed	Review progress with relatedness across all relationships in his life. Consider having Bella join in some sessions to discuss Tommy's progress and areas of need

(continued)

Table 8.2 (continued)

Primary Goods *Indicate priorities	Interventions		
	Short term: 3 months	Medium term: 6 months	Long term: 1 year or more
Inner peace **	Tommy will use the initial months of his treatment to explore options for finding inner peace that don't rely on sex or substance use. This can include progressive muscle relaxation, mindfulness, meditation, tai chi, yoga, etc.	Tommy will devote a period of time each day to one or more activities. He will use therapy to review his practices, including during this devoted time and also in daily life as needed (for example, practicing mindfulness while stuck in traffic)	Tommy can continue to review his progress in this area with his treatment team. Because the topic is not overly personal, he can consider developing a presentation on what he learns to benefit others in the treatment program
Mastery in work **	Identify job skills needed to obtain more secure and gainful employment	Use therapy to review and practice skills related to employment. Establish plan for getting periodic feedback from Tommy's employer	Review progress in employment and employer feedback. Review progress at upskilling and seeking out opportunities for growth
Community	Explore activities that bring Tommy closer to the community around him. This may include leisure activities or civic organizations that promote the public good (such as organized helping of neighbors)	Become involved in one or more community activities. Review necessary skills in therapy, using role plays and other methods to acquire and rehearse skills	Review progress and what Tommy has learned to continue building ties to the community around him
Mastery in play	Explore activities that Tommy can engage in on his own and with others that provide relief from the other expectations and obligations that Tommy has throughout the week	Develop a repertoire of leisure activities. Tommy is interested in cooking and playing guitar. Review progress in therapy, using role plays and other methods to acquire and rehearse skills	Review progress and what Tommy has learned to continue developing his capacities in this area
Creativity	Explore things that Tommy can do at home and at work that are new and extend his comfort zone. This can include playing his guitar in front of others and cooking new meals for Bella and his family	Tommy can review his progress in therapy, celebrating the victories he has in this area	As with other PHGs, Tommy can review progress and what Tommy has learned to continue developing his capacities in this area

(continued)

Table 8.2 (continued)

Primary Goods *Indicate priorities	Interventions		
	Short term: 3 months	Medium term: 6 months	Long term: 1 year or more
Knowledge	Tommy can do additional study on daily-life and relationship skills in order to bolster his skills. Tommy can also develop plans for continuing education depending on timing and availability of opportunities	Tommy can review his progress in therapy and get feedback from his treatment team. He can then use therapy to make adjustments to his knowledge acquisition accordingly.	As with other PHGs, Tommy can review progress and what Tommy has learned to continue developing his capacities in this area. Tommy and his team can also celebrate progress as it occurs
States of happiness and pleasure	Tommy can schedule time to do things that give him (and Bella) pleasure or simply make him/them happy in the moment. This might be as simple as making a nice dessert after dinner or going out to a movie	Tommy can review his progress in therapy, including how he manages his schedule with respect to activities that give him (alone, or with Bella) happiness and pleasure	As with other PHGs, Tommy can review progress and what Tommy has learned to continue developing his capacities in this area. Tommy and his team can also celebrate progress as it occurs
Spirituality	Tommy can use therapy to explore and discover who he is and what things give him a sense of meaning and purpose. Tommy can explore possible spiritual paths to see what, if anything, might be a good fit for him	Tommy can review what has and hasn't worked for him. He will be invited to discuss what he has learned and what steps he may wish to take in the future	Tommy can review progress and what Tommy has learned in order to continue developing his sense of fulfillment in this area

highway restaurant job to start a more stable one that provided him with greater opportunities and a decent salary. It contributed to his eventually getting out of poverty. He eventually stopped his cannabis use because he felt more inner peace by practicing the skills in his intervention plan and reflecting on his progress in building stable relationships at home and in the workplace. He found a dog for his family and concluded through caring for it that he was better able to learn than he had thought. Tommy eventually learned to speak about his needs instead of using destructive means. This was only possible after his efforts at developing better living conditions and more stable relationships.

After Tommy was in treatment for just under a year, he was discharged from treatment and sought supportive counseling in his community as a means for consolidating his gains and reviewing his progress in his life.

8.3 Linda[2]

8.3.1 Introduction

Linda is 42. She was arrested for arson after setting fire to the house she lived in with her partner, John. Fortunately, no one was hurt in this fire. She subsequently explained that she had many frustrations in her life and relationship and was motivated by despair and revenge to commit this crime. She wanted him to see the pain he had caused by leaving her. Although she sometimes made statements to the effect that he deserved it, Linda was heartbroken in the wake of her relationship problems. Linda has a full-scale IQ of 69 and has been described by previous therapists as having very little resilience. However, she is very clearly motivated to make changes in her life, is pleasant to speak with, and gets along well with others in her current surroundings.

8.3.2 Background Information

Linda grew up with her mother and father. She has an older sister and younger brother. Her mother had many medical problems that prevented her from working. Her father has diagnoses of bipolar disorder and gambling addiction. In her earliest years, Linda often witnessed aggression from her father toward her mother. Linda has now lost contact with her father and her brother. Her contact with her sister and mother is variable. During her adolescence, Linda became addicted to illegal drugs. From the ages of 16–23, she used heroin and methadone. Afterwards, she met a man named Dirk and became addicted to alcohol. Linda had two children with Dirk. During her pregnancies, Linda was able to stop drinking. However, her third pregnancy ended in miscarriage. Linda became overwhelmed by emotions and lacked the ability to manage them. She turned to excessive alcohol consumption to avoid these emotions. With the support of Dirk and the will to be able to take care of her children, Linda managed to stop drinking. After some time, Dirk found work and Linda relapsed again. She found herself lost in the use of alcohol, cannabis, and Valium. Dirk came to believe that a worthwhile relationship with Linda was not possible and left. Linda suddenly found herself as a single mother.

At those times when she was sober, Linda received ample support from her sister and mother. During those times of relapse into substance abuse, she experienced her interactions with them as very judgmental, making Linda feel inferior and avoid contact. Over time, she became increasingly estranged from her family, in large part

[2] We would like to sincerely thank Leen De Neve and Suzan Laureys (both affiliated to *Outreach De Steiger, Psychiatrisch Centrum Dr. Guislain*, Ghent, Belgium) who were involved in developing the case description of Linda.

because she lacked the skills for staying clean and sober and the ability to communicate in a way that might have kept her mother and sister closer.

Linda's life after Dirk's departure was marked by short-lived and often violent relationships, during which she was repeatedly the victim of partner violence. She also continued to use illegal substances. Her mental health suffered greatly as a result. In 1 year, Linda made three suicide attempts due to intoxication. She has not learned to talk about feelings, as her cognitive and emotional capabilities were too underdeveloped to deal with this. During one of her hospitalizations, Linda met John.

At the time of her arrest for arson, Linda and John had been together for 1 year. She was working on and off for a small business that cleaned homes and offices. The relationship was tumultuous, and both were engaged in problematic substance use. Linda and John were each terribly jealous, which, under the influence of alcohol and substances, often led to heated arguments. Such was the case on the day of the index offense. When John left the house during an argument, Linda proceeded to set fire to their mattress, which quickly spread to the curtains. Within only a short time, the house was a total loss. Linda was arrested by the police and stayed in jail pending her trial. Her children were placed in foster care. She explained to the police and others that she had a lot of frustration and a desire for revenge before committing this crime.

Immediately upon her arrest, Linda was sent to a jail to await processing in the legal system. Linda was found guilty. However, due to the nature of her intellectual disability (a full-scale IQ of 69 and considerable adaptive impairments) and her substance abuse disorder, the judge assigned a legal guardian to her and ordered her into an intensive residential home in lieu of incarceration. As long as she was active in treatment with no further criminal behavior, she could receive these services, which would provide supervised access to the community. If Linda was not able to manage her behavior and benefit from treatment, she would be sent to a special unit within the prison system.

8.3.3 Assessment

Once in the program, Linda participated in an assessment to identify her risks and needs. The evaluator used the Multi-Trajectory Theory of Adult Firesetting (M-TTAF; Gannon et al., 2012) as one means of understanding Linda's actions. The M-TAFF is "an integration of current theory, typological, and research knowledge into a comprehensive etiological theory of firesetting" (p. 2). The results of this assessment found that Linda's firesetting had occurred as part of an "emotionally expressive/need for recognition" trajectory. This meant that her actions were essentially a cry for help that was similar to actions taken by those who have been diagnosed with borderline personality disorder, had histories of self-harm, suicide attempts, and who frequently experience themselves as unrecognized, unheard, and unseen. Importantly, the M-TTAF indicated that Linda had not acted out of a sense of grievance, antisocial cognitions, or a specific interest in fire.

The evaluator used a number of other measures in the assessment process, but because of the dearth of validated measures for women primarily, they relied on clinical interviews and record reviews to gather clinically relevant information. The evaluator concluded that in the absence of more proven methodology, Linda was best described as being at low–moderate risk for firesetting and high risk for further substance abuse and self-harm. Further, Linda's risk for engaging in these behaviors would depend on the circumstances that she found herself in. Within the setting of her residential program, she could remain at low risk with the provision of effective services by trained staff.

A further review of Linda's life revealed several risk factors, many of which have been in place since her early years. Importantly, the evaluator (and subsequently, Linda's therapists) had been able to view each of these factors as reflecting dynamic processes across Linda's life. Fortunately, each of these is amenable to therapy:

- A history of substance dependence
- Self-regulation problems (including rapid escalating negative emotions)
- Antisocial cognitions
- Antisocial personality traits
- Few problem-solving skills, especially when upset, angry, or anxious
- Few hobbies or leisure interests
- Relationship instability
- Emotional loneliness

A simple list of risk factors is unhelpful for all but the most basic tasks of an assessment. Further, these risk factors emerged from research conducted almost exclusively on adult males. Useful questions in considering each risk factor would be: How does being female influence each of these factors? How has each factor played a role in her identity as a woman? As signaling devices (see Chap. 2), each of these risk factors is associated with PHGs that Linda has sought throughout her life, often beyond her awareness. Before exploring those further, a brief narrative case formulation might be helpful.

Linda had grown up in an environment that often couldn't and wouldn't support her growth and development as a girl and young woman. She was witness to family violence and suffered emotional neglect. She had little guidance to help her achieve developmental tasks. It is not surprising that she appeared to develop so little resilience. On the one hand, she developed skills for in-the-moment survival in dangerous environments (through substance abuse, being quick to anger and willing to fight back against perceived threats). On the other hand, this adaptation to her environment came at the expense of other vital life skills, including regulating emotions, anticipating problematic situations, and solving problems as they arose in her daily life.

For several years of her life, more traditional mental health professionals described Linda as an antisocial woman (she had made provocative statements such as, "I didn't mind he nearly burned into ashes"). Setting aside the highly pejorative nature of labels such as "antisocial," such statements are vague and do not point to a way forward. While labeling behaviors or conditions can assist in treatment planning, labeling the entire woman as antisocial not only misses the mark with respect to human complexity but only resulted in shame and reduced amenability to treatment.

8.3.4 GLM-Specific Assessment

Although being described as having antisocial cognitions and personality features, Linda's presentation in the program (which was more adapted to her needs) was more as a woman with limited emotional development, with difficulties in assessing situations and their consequences, having little insight into what others think or feel, and having underdeveloped coping skills for dealing with the stresses of daily life. The treatment team came to understand her as a person who cares deeply for others but faces many obstacles in building and sustaining relationships.

It is in the above context that her arson occurred. A combination of low tolerance for frustration, limited cognitive ability, feelings of needing to send a strong message, and anxiety around the loss of yet another relationship were some of the primary factors resulting in her offending. Her search for inner peace was through substance abuse, and the relationship with John was strongly connected with her own lack of agency and challenges with relatedness. She wanted to be loved but had little control over herself or the relationship because of its tumultuous nature.

Linda dreamed of stability for herself and her children. Her desire for a better future was strong, but she encountered internal and external obstacles as she attempted to build a new life for herself. Linda often feels that she is not good enough and fails in life. On several occasions in the past, she has tried to end her life. She felt that running away or numbing are not appropriate solutions to her problems, but she does not know of any other ways. She says she wants to learn this, but that the therapy sessions often trigger memories from the past in her. As a result, she increasingly avoids therapy. She slips into substance abuse again and again. It seems as if she can only find inner peace and a decrease in stress by fleeing into alcohol or suicide attempts.

Linda has a limited social network. Although she finds support from her mother and sister, there are moments of condemnation and rejection that distance her from them. Her children are currently the only stable relationships Linda has. She finds it important to be a good mother, and this role gives her a sense of purpose in life. Linda searches for relationships in which she feels supported and understood, but often encounters the wrong people in doing so. Linda indicated that she no longer wants a partner. She no longer wants all the problems that come with it.

As noted above, Linda reports that it is very difficult for her to be alone; she feels painful loneliness often. It is very difficult for Linda to manage her boundaries, both with family, fellow patients, partners, and social workers. Linda struggles to discuss this. Professionals and friends have often felt that they must drag this out of Linda. On the one hand, Linda wants to express her boundaries better, and on the other, she does not want to hurt anyone. As a result, she lets others overstep her boundaries and often finds herself in unsafe situations.

In summary, PHGs that are particularly important to Linda include:

- Relatedness (close relationships and friendships)
- Agency (autonomy and independence)
- Inner peace (freedom from emotional turmoil without relapsing to substance abuse)
- Life (living and surviving)
- States of happiness and pleasure (without relapsing to substance abuse)
- Spirituality (a sense of meaning and purpose in her life; in Linda's case, her identity as a mother)

PHGs that are less important to Linda include:

- Mastery in work
- Mastery in play (leisure activities)
- Community
- Knowledge (particularly with respect to learning about herself, her relationships, and job opportunities)
- Creativity

PHGs that are implicated in Linda's offending include:

- Life (her survival instincts have led to behavioral patterns that brought her into conflict with the law and with other PHGs). This is reflected in her risk factors of:
  - Emotional dysregulation
  - Problems with coping
  - Diminished skills for anticipating and solving problems
  - Aggressive acts toward others
- Relatedness. This is reflected in her risk factors of:
  - Relationship instability
  - Attitudes supportive of antisocial behavior
- Inner peace. This is reflected in her risk factors of:
  - Substance abuse
  - Rapid escalating negative emotions
- States of happiness and pleasure (via substance abuse)
- Knowledge (lacking the skills to prevent problematic behavior generally)

Obstacles to the Primary Human Goods Involved in Linda's Offense

Across her life, Linda's pursuit of the PHGs showed that the coherence of her implicit GLP was almost entirely vertical. She prioritized some PHGs at the expense of others, resulting in a GLP that also lacked horizontal coherence; her attempts to secure PHGs were not well integrated. Throughout her life, Linda had either been unable or unready to develop a GLP in which the PHGs would cohere and be integrated.

Finally, Linda had faced many obstacles to building a GLP. Initially, Linda had grown up in a chaotic family environment and now lived in an environment that offered her few opportunities (external capacity). As she grew, she developed very few skills for managing her daily life successfully (internal capacity). Having grown up in adversity, she developed a very narrow scope to her implicit GLP, focusing primarily on short-sighted efforts in the PHGs of life, relationships, inner peace, and states of happiness and pleasure. These efforts were short-sighted in the sense that while they may have helped Linda in the present moment, they were unlikely to be effective in the long term. Not surprisingly, her need for inner peace and states of happiness and pleasure, which she attained through drugs and alcohol, came into direct conflict with her relationships with others (conflict between both PHGs and the means to attain them). When it appeared that John was leaving her due to her drug use, she resorted to inappropriate means by setting the fire that resulted in her arrest. In Linda's case, this resulted in a sequence along the lines of:

- Problems with external capacity
- Problems with internal capacity
- Narrow scope
- Conflict between goods and means
- Use of inappropriate means

This sequence of obstacles would be important for Linda's therapists to understand. It would have been easy for programs to become preoccupied with Linda's lack of internal capacity and want to immediately initiate a skills-based curricula. By understanding the after-effects of Linda's adversity (problems with both internal and external capacity), the staff could eventually better understand Linda's narrowed scope and conflict between goods and means. This illustrates the value of viewing DRFs as signaling devices that point to specific motivational systems and their associated PHG, and challenges in achieving valued goals in adaptive and personally satisfying ways.

Linda's practical identity (see Chap. 1) revolved around her most highly prized PHGs of relatedness and spirituality (in particular, her experience of motherhood). At the time that she set the fire, each of these had become nearly impossible. It is therefore not surprising that her life seemed bleak, and she was grief-stricken at the time she set the fire.

8.3.5 *Good Lives Model Mapping Tool*

As a final step in the assessment phase, the evaluator worked with Linda to explore her good life plan (GLP) at the time of her firesetting. Their work on this appears below (Table 8.3):

Table 8.3 Linda's mapping table

Primary goods	Importance	Means	Internal strengths	Internal obstacles	External strengths	External obstacles	Relationship to offending
Life	High (but variable depending on mood and circumstances)	Has required public assistance with housing; has viewed relationships as key to survival	Motivated to stay safe in housing and provide for children	Prone to emotional collapse and dysregulation; intellectual disability; substance abuse	Variable depending on nature of relationships with family and lovers	Financial problems	At times she believes she may not be able to survive, she has resorted to self-harm, suicide attempts, firesetting, and substance abuse
Relatedness	High	Attempts to maintain family contacts; attempts to keep partners in her life (although these were rarely successful)	High motivation to maintain relationships; loyalty to those she loves	Lack of relationship skills (such as the ability to manage boundaries); emotional dysregulation; tendency to idealize relationships only to be disappointed	A committed treatment team; mother and sister wish for her successful rehabilitation	Recent losses of significant relationships. Lack of available potential partners	The emotional collapse and dysregulation that resulted from losing relationships was a primary motivator in Linda's firesetting

(continued)

Table 8.3 (continued)

Primary goods	Importance	Means	Internal strengths	Internal obstacles	External strengths	External obstacles	Relationship to offending
Community	Low	The closest that Linda came to achieving this PHG was in seeing herself as part of the community of those involved with substance abuse	Linda was not focused on this PHG at the time of her offense. However, Linda is motivated to get along with others and to fit into her surroundings	Linda was preoccupied with substance abuse and her lost relationships and did not focus on this PHG	There were community resources at the time of her offending that would have been available to her and will be in the future	Linda's track record of substance abuse meant that she was viewed with suspicion by her community	This PHG played an indirect role in Linda's offending. Had she taken advantage of community resources and programming, she would have been less likely to commit her crimes
Mastery in work	Low	In lieu of pursuing this goal, Linda relied on her partners	Linda had previously enjoyed keeping herself busy and active	Linda had few work skills and possessed little motivation to work, due to self-limiting beliefs, including shame. Her low IQ also made employment a challenge	Linda resided in an area where jobs and the opportunity to upskill were available	Local schools and employers were very wary of hiring someone with her historical behaviors and intellectual disability	This PHG played an indirect role in Linda's offending, in that had she sought the stability of gainful employment, she may have been less likely to engage in substance abuse and firesetting

Mastery in play	Moderate	Linda used drugs and alcohol in the pursuit of this PHG	Linda had previously enjoyed keeping herself busy and active	Linda confused the acts of taking drugs and drinking alcohol with mastery experiences in recreation.	Linda's community offered diverse opportunities for recreation.	Linda's family and partners appear to have been unsuccessful in helping her to achieve this PHG without the use of drugs and alcohol	Linda's substance abuse had a disinhibiting effect on Linda and did not help her decision-making with respect to the fire that she set
Creativity	Moderate	Linda's primary means for this PHG was in finding and using drugs and alcohol	Linda has always enjoyed having new experiences.	Linda has only been able to have new experiences through substance abuse and forming new relationships	Linda's community offered diverse opportunities for creative endeavors.	Many possible community resources were off-limits because they were not welcoming of Linda	On its own, this PHG contributed very little to Linda's crime beyond the fact that the drugs she took interfered with her judgment with respect to her crime of firesetting

(continued)

Table 8.3 (continued)

Primary goods	Importance	Means	Internal strengths	Internal obstacles	External strengths	External obstacles	Relationship to offending
Agency	High	Whatever the physical aspects of addiction, Linda viewed substance abuse as a choice she could make independently	Linda has pursued some form of agency throughout her life despite her high level of commitment to her relationships. This has been most evident in her engaging in behaviors that run counter to the wishes of her family and-Partners	Linda's emotional and physical dependence on substance use and her various partners has been a very strong obstacle to achieving this goal	Linda's family and partners would be very supportive of her taking more responsibility for her own agency	Within the pursuit of her lifestyle to date, Linda saw few opportunities to engage in prosocial acts of agency	Linda's firesetting was, among other things, a result of the pursuit of agency at a time when she was angry and heartbroken at the loss of a relationship and wanting to call attention to herself and her needs
Knowledge	Low		Linda's attempts to gain knowledge tended to be driven by momentary needs, and therefore not a prime focus for her. When motivated by her relationships, she could be quick to seek out knowledge of others' activities, etc.	Linda's full-scale IQ of 69 acted as a strong internal obstacle	Linda's schools and family were highly motivated to help her receive an education	Linda's schools and family were not adequately resourced to help Linda in this area	This PHG played a role in Linda's firesetting, in that the pursuit of knowledge around emotional regulation skills would have helped prevent this crime

Inner peace	High	Linda turned to drugs and alcohol, as well as her relationships, in the hopes that they would help her to find a sense of inner peace	Linda had a strong motivation to achieve this PHG. However, Linda lacked the skills to find inner peace without relying on drugs, alcohol, and her relationships with others	Linda's use of drugs and alcohol was self-limiting and did not bring her inner peace in the long run. Instead, it prevented her from developing longer-term skills in this area	Resources for overcoming these internal obstacles and helping Linda to develop emotional regulation skills and other sources of inner peace are plentiful in the community	People in Linda's community often struggled to understand her and provide her with the assistance that she needed	This PHG played a direct role in Linda's firesetting. Had she had more skills for emotional self-regulation, it likely would not have occurred at all
States of happiness and pleasure	High	Linda turned to drugs and alcohol, as well as her relationships, in the hopes that they would help her to find momentary states of happiness and pleasure in an otherwise challenging life	As with the PHG of inner peace, Linda had a strong motivation to achieve this PHG. However, Linda lacked the skills to find these states without relying on drugs, alcohol, and her relationships with others	Linda's acquisition of happiness and pleasure through drugs, alcohol did not serve her well in the long run, as evidenced by their effects on her relationships	As with the PHG of inner peace, resources for overcoming these internal obstacles and helping Linda to find these states are plentiful in the community	People in Linda's community often disapproved of her behavior and didn't provide her with the assistance that she needed to achieve this PHG differently.	Linda did not set the fire in order to experience pleasure. She might have been happy had others seen it as the cry for help that she felt it was

(continued)

Table 8.3 (continued)

Primary goods	Importance	Means	Internal strengths	Internal obstacles	External strengths	External obstacles	Relationship to offending
Spirituality	Moderate	Linda has gained a sense of meaning and purpose through her relationships with others. When these relationships have failed, the effects have been along the lines of an existential crisis for her	Linda has long been motivated to understand who she is and what her place is in the world. She desires to be the best mother that she can be	Linda's behaviors have often resulted in confusion about how she fits into the world around her	There are numerous resources in the community for Linda to explore with respect to spirituality	Some opportunities for spiritual development will be closed off to Linda due to her past behaviors	Linda's firesetting may have had an indirect contribution to this PHG in that she has had a long history of uncertainty as to who she is in the world and within her relationships. This could be explored further in treatment

8.3.6 GLM Intervention

Following her assessment, Linda began the treatment program. She attended group therapy sessions and found connection with other group members. Linda had long dreamed of a new home for herself and her children. She had planned to rebuild her life without a partner (at least for the foreseeable future), fearing that relationships would only cause further problems. She also wanted to get a job that built on her previous part-time experiences of cleaning homes and offices. In the larger picture, she wanted to be among people and be part of society. When opportunities appeared that could help her reach her own goals (for example, others starting up a thrift store and inviting her to help), Linda often dropped out. She would not attend external appointments, despite encouragement or guidance from her treatment team. At one point, Linda eloped from the program for several days and started drinking again to forget her problems. She returned to the program on her own, narrowly averting imprisonment.

Because Linda came across as strong and capable, fellow patients frequently told her their problems. Linda could not help but try to solve these problems for them at such times. However, she was often unsuccessful at this, which led to her becoming overwhelmed and believing herself to be a failure not worthy of anything good in life. Linda clearly had high expectations for herself and believed that everything she did should be immediately successful; to her, there was no room for trial and error. She would rather not try than make a mistake. When this happens, the only way out Linda could see is to turn to alcohol.

Linda and her treatment team worked together to develop a GLM intervention plan. At first, she first questioned some of the proposals put forward by team members, indicating that she did not feel comfortable doing so. As a result, Linda and the team worked together to clarify steps to shape the plan into something she felt motivated to follow. The results appear below (Table 8.4). The initial steps focused on opportunities and challenges inside the institution, while subsequent steps included a focus on how Linda could eventually integrate into the community.

The treatment team, along with Linda, next agreed that providing a treatment specific to her traumatic experiences would help not only in resolving her experiences, but because it would also help her attain virtually all the PHGs. By learning about how much of her life had been a response to her early life adversity, she could better work toward a more balanced and self-determined lifestyle. The pain and the consequences of these memories motivate Linda to give it a chance. She began a course of eye movement desensitization and reprocessing (EMDR; Shapiro, 2018) to minimize the effect of these experiences as an obstacle to reaching inner peace. Linda reported that this was quite successful and enabled her to work more diligently in other areas.

While in the treatment program, Linda discovered an interest in writing. She joined the editorial board of the newsletter of the activity center of the psychiatric clinic, using her existing strengths involving knowledge about different subjects. She enjoyed writing about them and realized when interviewing other patients that

Table 8.4 Linda's GLM intervention plan

Primary goods *Indicate priorities	Interventions		
	Short term: 3 months	Medium term: 6 months	Long term: 1 year or more
Life *	Trauma therapy to examine her past experiences attempting to work toward this PHG Education and skills training for independent living. Education around substance abuse disorders; introduction to support groups	Continue trauma therapy as needed, with a focus on safety planning in the future Independent living skills rehearsal and refinement, with discussion of how some skills are implemented in the community Linda can participate in ongoing support groups such as alcoholics anonymous and narcotics anonymous	Continued review of independent living skills, with safety planning as necessary in preparation for gradual community reintegration Continue using support groups to help manage urges or temptations related to drugs and alcohol
Relatedness*	Trauma therapy to address early life relational adversity. Education around relationship skillsLinda can also examine her daily interactions with staff as a means to explore relationship skills Linda's interviewing people for the newsletter can also help to inspire learning in this area	Linda can use program activities and therapy sessions to acquire and rehearse interpersonal skills, with a goal of experiencing herself as competent in a broader range of relationships Linda can continue to interview people as a means to build skills in relatedness	Linda can continue to use therapy to address progress in building, maintaining, and strengthening her relationships with others
Agency *	Trauma therapy to help understand how adverse experiences in her life have interfered with her working toward increased agency Continue discussions started in assessment around living independently and free of being dependent on men	Acquire and rehearse independent living skills Use therapy to address building a self-determined lifestyle that does not require the support of men	Linda can engage in an increasing number of community activities (including work and educational experiences) on her own and/or with staff members nearby but not closely supervising her Linda can then review her experiences in therapy

(continued)

Table 8.4 (continued)

Primary goods *Indicate priorities	Interventions		
	Short term: 3 months	Medium term: 6 months	Long term: 1 year or more
Inner peace *	A primary focus of Linda's treatment will be in developing emotional regulation skills. Linda can use the first months of treatment to learn about these skills and to participate in trauma therapy, which will prepare her for creating longer lasting capacities in this area Linda will be introduced to possible methods for attaining a sense of inner peace, such as through mindfulness and meditation. Linda can use canine-assisted therapy as an adjunct treatment to help in this area	Linda can use therapy to develop and rehearse emotional regulation skills. She can use experiences from her days in the program to explore what has and hasn't worked well for her and get feedback from others Linda can continue to use program and community resources to explore means for achieving inner peace Linda can use canine-assisted therapy as an adjunct treatment to help in this area	Linda can continue to focus on using skills for emotional regulation and finding states of being free from emotional turmoil in the community as well as in the program
States of happiness and pleasure *	Linda can use support groups to learn from others how they gain happiness and experience pleasure without the use of drugs or alcohol	Linda can learn and practice skills for experiencing happiness and pleasure in the program	Linda can learn and practice skills for experiencing happiness and pleasure in the community as well as the program
Community	Linda can use supervised activities in the community to rehearse skills and learn about resources. She can then discuss what she's learned with staff members on her return	Linda can be provided with supervised employment, as well as opportunities for upskilling	Linda can work in the community with staff nearby as a safety measure Linda can also take classes in the community as a means of exploring options that are available to her there

(continued)

Table 8.4 (continued)

Primary goods *Indicate priorities	Interventions		
	Short term: 3 months	Medium term: 6 months	Long term: 1 year or more
Mastery in work	Linda can learn job skills within the program through a supervised employment experience. She can use therapy and her work with the newsletter to explore what employment she is best suited for	Linda can seek out a job in a setting where she can be supervised, at first, to ensure that she can be successful	Linda can work in the community and use therapy to explore her successes and shortcomings
Mastery in play	Linda can engage in recreational activities to explore her likes and dislikes and to build on activities in which she experiences competence	Linda can continue to explore and engage in recreational activities that she likes with a focus on activities in which she experiences competence	Linda can engage in recreational activities in the community and with community groups of people with similar interests
Creativity	Linda can take classes in writing and poetry, as well as exploring other areas of creative endeavor within the program	Linda will be encouraged to schedule time in her week to try new creative endeavors in addition to her writing efforts	Linda can seek out and engage in community activities to focus on creative endeavors or to simply try new things
Knowledge	Linda can work with educational staff in the program to understand her learning style and begin work on completing her education The staff can also teach Linda fire safety skills as one part of her treatment for firesetting Linda can also work to learn about her areas of interest, including writing	Linda can continue to take classes to complete her education and continue studying her areas of interest, including writing In line with other therapeutic activities, Linda can work with her therapist to create a safety plan for fire use to help with learning how to manage any impulses, should they occur Linda can also continue to study writing	Linda can continue her education by taking classes in the community

(continued)

Table 8.4 (continued)

Primary goods *Indicate priorities	Interventions		
	Short term: 3 months	Medium term: 6 months	Long term: 1 year or more
Spirituality	Linda can use therapy to explore who she is. This includes her identity as a woman, a family member, and a mother. She can use therapy to explore how she fits into the world around her, and what activities give her a sense of meaning and purpose Linda can also explore what kinds of spiritual pathways might be missing from her life that she would like to pursue	Linda can continue to explore what aspects of her life give her a sense of meaning and purpose. She can review what does and doesn't work for her in the program	Linda can be given access to activities that will boost her sense of spirituality in the community as well as the program

she also wanted to learn to talk about and deal with her feelings. To find some peace and stability, it was important to Linda that she no longer avoid her emotions. Addressing these would also enhance her self-esteem. However, she didn't feel safe addressing emotional content most of the time. Through creative therapy and canine-assisted interventions, she learned to talk about and experience feelings through expressive forms and in relation to the dog she worked with. She experienced a deeper sense of agency and being good at something as a result.

Before too long, Linda addressed her issues with substance abuse and dependence. She learned to reach out to others when it is difficult to remain sober. Family therapy with her mother and sister led to the opportunity to speak with them when experiencing this difficulty. Because she learnt how to talk with others before relapsing, her mother and sister began to recognize her emerging competencies, especially when they were supporting her. They want to assist her in her recovery process and are willing to do what they can. By working toward the goods of relatedness and agency in this way (by including Linda's most important community supports), she is more effective at preventing substance abuse.

To support her in assuming her maternal role, which she felt was a significant portion of the purpose of her life (the PHG of spirituality) and a significant part of her practical identity, Linda became involved in parental counseling. Together with a therapist, Linda made a game box so she could play with the children during their visits, with the twofold goal of strengthening the bond with them and strengthening her parenting skills, especially as her children grow and change. As she develops these skills, relying on erstwhile antisocial cognitions, attitudes, and beliefs became less desirable.

Because Linda had never lived independently (without parents or partner) before, her team employed a form of skills training aimed at equipping her with the skills to live independently (for example, housekeeping and cooking) along with basic administration such as paying bills. Linda was enthusiastic about this because it started with cooking, something she was highly motivated to do. This increased her sense of agency and helped her reach a goal of an independent life with her children. This, in turn, increased her motivation for treatment in general.

As a result of this increased motivation, Linda became ready to focus on other meaningful activities. She began to work in a thrift store. In this environment, with the support of a social work paraprofessional, she learned how to sort and value clothing. Her opportunities once again increased for meeting new people, connecting, becoming good at something and having more control over her life, including an income that allows her to live independently. It also helped reduce another risk factor: problematic spending of free time.

Linda's case became a textbook example of the importance of designing treatment around what is meaningful and important to the client. While many treatment programs would consider job skills and trauma treatment to be ancillary and not necessarily related to risk, in Linda's case, these comprehensive approaches gave her important life skills, increased her motivation to succeed, and ultimately helped her to attain the twin goals of manage risks and enhancing her well-being.

References

Andrews, D., Bonta, J., & Wormith, J. S. (n.d.). *Level of service/case management inventory (LS/CMI™) [Database record]*. APA PsycTests. https://doi.org/10.1037/t05029-000

Gannon, T. A., Ciardha, C. Ó., Doley, R. M., & Alleyne, E. (2012). The multi-trajectory theory of adult firesetting (M-TTAF). *Aggression and Violent Behavior, 17*(2), 107–121. https://doi.org/10.1016/j.avb.2011.08.001

Hart, S. D., & Boer, D. P. (2021). Structured professional judgment guidelines for sexual violence risk assessment: The sexual violence risk-20 (SVR-20) versions 1 and 2 and risk for sexual violence protocol (RSVP). In K. S. Douglas & R. K. Otto (Eds.), *Handbook of violence risk assessment* (2nd ed., pp. 322–358). Routledge/Taylor & Francis Group. https://doi.org/10.4324/9781315518374-18

Kelley, S. M., Willis, G. M., & Thornton, D. (2022). Clinical applications of the Structured Assessment of PROtective Factors against Sexual Offending (SAPROF-SO), version 1. *Journal of Sexual Aggression, 28*(3), 377–392. https://doi.org/10.1080/13552600.2021.2020345

Shapiro, F. (2018). *Eye movement desensitization and reprocessing (EMDR) therapy: Basic principles, protocols, and procedures* (3rd ed.). Guilford Press.

Chapter 9
Empirical Support for the GLM as a Rehabilitation Theory

9.1 Introduction

Is the good lives model (GLM) practice framework empirically supported? Do interventions derived from it demonstrate effectiveness in terms of promoting desistance from crime? Crime is costly, and preventing repeat offending requires investment in rehabilitation and reintegration initiatives with demonstrated empirical support. Pouring resources into ineffective services and programs risks increasing the personal, social, and economic costs associated with crime. Sexual and violent offending, in particular, carry incalculable costs to individuals, families, and communities. Accordingly, decades of research in criminology and correctional/forensic psychology have sought to answer the question of what works to reduce the likelihood of reoffending. An impetus behind the development of the GLM was to advance research through offering an alternative rehabilitation framework to approaches that focused almost exclusively on recidivism reduction, potentially at the cost of engaging clients in the process of change. Unlike medical interventions, effective psychological interventions require a therapeutic relationship characterized by warmth, empathy, and praise (e.g., Norcross, 2002). Indeed, it's unlikely that clients can change simply through being passive recipients of a rehabilitation program.

Most of the "what works" literature in correctional psychology has focused on the risk, need, and responsivity (RNR) principles of correctional interventions (Bonta & Andrews, 2024). Numerous meta-analyses and systematic reviews have found support for the RNR principles, although a recent umbrella review of the RNR's evidence base drew attention to the poor quality of underlying research (Fazel et al., 2024). With that caveat, offending treatment programs that tailor intensity based on recidivism risk, focus on empirically identified criminogenic needs, and are delivered using empirically supported treatment models (e.g., Cognitive Behavioral Therapy; CBT) are more effective—at least in terms of recidivism

T. Ward et al., *The Good Lives Model of Correctional Rehabilitation*,
Advances in Preventing and Treating Violence and Aggression,
https://doi.org/10.1007/978-3-031-95559-4_9

outcomes—than those programs that fail to adhere to one or more of the RNR principles (Bonta & Andrews, 2024; Hanson et al., 2009). In addition, consistent input from registered psychologists is associated with improved treatment effectiveness (Gannon et al., 2019). In the early days of the GLM, the extent to which the GLM added value to the RNR principles and CBT was debated emphatically between RNR proponents and GLM practitioners (Andrews et al., 2011; Bonta & Andrews, 2003; Ward et al., 2012; Wormith et al., 2012). Retrospectively, it seems there was no need to position the GLM and RNR against each other. More than two decades later, these debates hold little relevance to current research and practice. Indeed, GLM-informed programs can (and should) accommodate RNR principles. Nevertheless, in our collective efforts to promote more humanistic, strengths-based approaches to correctional rehabilitation—the most common criticism is the lack of empirical support for GLM-derived rehabilitation programs. Scientist practitioners will appreciate the need for advancing the GLM's evidence base, and so, the aim of this chapter is to take stock of extant research and inspire ongoing research.

The empirical adequacy of a practice framework can be explored in numerous ways, including examining a theory's underlying etiological assumptions and then testing interventions derived from it against interventions with known empirical support. Thus, the empirical adequacy of the GLM can be examined through evaluating its knowledge-related assumptions and the effectiveness of GLM-informed interventions relative to those adhering to RNR principles. This chapter will begin by reviewing empirical research examining the knowledge-related assumptions set out in Chap. 1, followed by a review of nascent research on the effectiveness of GLM-informed correctional interventions. The chapter will highlight key gaps in the GLM's evidence base and conclude with some proposals for future research.

9.2 Empirical Research Examining Knowledge-Related Assumptions of the GLM

Mallion et al. (2020) conducted a systematic review of GLM assumptions (and interventions, reviewed in the next section), identifying 12 relevant studies. These studies focused on testing the assumptions that offending reflects an attempt to fulfill one or more primary human goods (PHGs) and that obstacles in a good life plan (GLP) prevent prosocial attainment of PHGs. The review found some support related to the former assumption; however, divergent approaches to assessing PHGs (e.g., interview questions aligned with each PHG vs. general quality of life questionnaires) likely contributed to overall mixed findings. They also found support for the latter assumption, although no studies in their review considered the obstacles of conflict and scope. The following is an overview of selected studies from Mallion et al.'s review, alongside research published since then, with the aim of illustrating the scope of extant research examining the GLM's knowledge-related assumptions. The primary focus here is on studies with adult samples. Four studies with adolescent samples were included in Mallion et al.'s review (Barendregt, 2015; Barendregt et al., 2018; Chu et al., 2015; Van Damme et al., 2016), and at least one study with an adolescent sample has been published since (Appiah & Billen, 2024).

Early studies explored the application of the GLM with adults convicted of sexual offenses. In the first such study, Purvis (2005, 2010) interviewed 26 participants, finding states of happiness and pleasure, relatedness, inner peace, mastery in play, agency, and life were pursued directly through sexual offending. In another study, Willis and Grace (2008) retrospectively examined release plan quality between adult men previously imprisoned for sexual offending who subsequently reoffended (n = 39) and a group matched for static risk and time since release who did not (n = 42). They included a variable intended to capture whether release plans contained concrete approach-oriented goals (i.e., secondary goods) that aligned with one or more PHGs. Such goals were more common in release planning for participants who did not reoffend, compared to those who did, suggesting prosocial attainment of PHGs may have protected against recidivism. Willis and Ward (2011) later explored the importance of PHGs and relationships between reentry experiences and PHG attainment with 16 adult men living in the community following imprisonment for a sexual offense. They found that the majority of participants considered most PHGs were at least moderately important in their lives and that positive reentry experiences (i.e., considering access to accommodation, social support, and employment—all associated with external capacity to attain PHGs) were associated with increased goods attainment 6 months post-release.

A handful of studies have examined GLM assumptions as they relate to nonsexual offending. Mallion (2021) examined knowledge-related assumptions of the GLM in the context of street gang membership. Using a sample of incarcerated individuals (N = 30, n = 17 involved in street gangs), they found street gang membership afforded means for attaining the full range of PHGs. As examples, gang members attained life through financial gain to secure basic needs and protection from harm. They found states of happiness and pleasure through substance misuse and access to sexual relationships. Agency came in the form of status and respect afforded by gang membership. Community manifested through a sense of belonging. Mastery in work was attained through "deviant entrepreneurship" (p. 300), knowledge took the form of learning to offend. Members found relatedness through close friendships with gang peers. Moreover, they found support for each of the four obstacles to goods attainment: PHGs were sought through gang membership when prosocial methods were unavailable or inaccessible, often due to unemployment, poor academic achievement, and community disorganization (problems with external capacity). Difficulties with emotional regulation and expression were identified as problems with internal capacity. A disregard of primary goods and a resulting lack of scope in an individual's GLP was linked with offending for some participants (e.g., a lack of self-care—relevant to the PHG of life—increasing willingness to expose oneself to dangerous situations). Experiences of conflict between goods and/or means were commonly observed (e.g., engagement in territorial behavior in pursuit of community impacting attainment of inner peace).

Taylor (2017) interviewed 30 individuals with a combined total of 353 residential burglary convictions in the 4 years prior to interview, and a total lifetime self-report estimate of more than 3394 residential burglaries. Interviews aimed to explore perceived reasons for the onset and continuity of offending with the GLM applied during data analysis. The primary motivation for offending across all but one participant was the primary good of life. Residential burglary meant obtaining money to secure accommodation and basic subsistence. A notable obstacle toward prosocial attainment of life was unemployment, with all participants being unemployed when committing most of their offenses. Knowledge and mastery also appeared in that several participants regarded themselves as "experts" in burglary, skilled in navigating security systems, and carrying out their crimes quietly and methodologically to avoid detection. Agency was simultaneously achieved and threatened: sometimes achieved through burglary, yet the threat of losing agency through imprisonment was also seen as a risk or "occupational hazard" (pg. 443). States of happiness and pleasure were obtained through offending itself, providing a buzz, as well as through monetary rewards that were often used to fund hedonistic and/or exuberant lifestyles.

A small number of studies have explored knowledge-related assumptions with general community samples. Loney and Harkins (2018) examined knowledge-related assumptions with a student sample ($N = 340$). Participants generally endorsed the importance of all PHGs, and specific correlations were found between the use of maladaptive strategies to attain selected PHGs (e.g., manipulating others to achieve agency), and self-reported offending. Specifically, the use of maladaptive strategies to seek agency and inner peace was predictive of violent offending, maladaptive strategies to seek inner peace and states of happiness and pleasure predicted drug-related offending, and maladaptive strategies to achieve agency predicted acquisitive offending. More recently, Olson et al. (2024) examined etiological assumptions of the GLM in a representative community sample of 1484 adults living in the USA. Through factor analysis, the authors developed a 45-item good lives assessment of domains (GLAD) scale to assess perceptions of life satisfaction across the GLM's 11 PHGs. Items were rated on a five-point Likert-type scale to indicate agreement with statements such as "I am free to make my own choices" (agency), "My emotions don't overwhelm me" (inner peace), "On most days, I enjoy the way my life is going" (states of happiness and pleasure), and "I can achieve or keep optimal physical health" (life), with higher scores indicative of higher satisfaction. Overall, GLAD scores were higher for participants who self-reported no engagement in crime or deviance in the preceding 12 months compared to those participants who reported engagement in crime or deviance.

Collectively, the reviewed studies provide general preliminary support for core knowledge-related assumptions of the GLM. Across varied samples, there is evidence that offending behavior relates to the purposeful pursuit of one or more PHGs in the context of limited capacity for seeking underlying goods in prosocial ways. The practice implications of the GLM therefore have some empirical grounding. Next, we turn our attention to empirical evaluations of interventions influenced by, or derived from, the GLM (also see Willis & Ward, 2024).

9.3 Empirical Support for the Effectiveness of GLM-Informed Interventions

Applied appropriately, GLM-derived interventions adhere to each of the RNR principles, embedding them within a broader strengths-based practice framework. It can be argued that the large body of empirical literature supporting the RNR also supports the GLM. In short, the GLM retains the merits of the RNR while addressing its limitations, especially difficulties motivating and engaging clients in the rehabilitation process (Mann, 2000; Ward & Maruna, 2007; Yates, 2009). It does so through supporting prosocial acquisition of valued PHGs, which requires addressing risk-relevant propensities conceptualized in the GLM as problems with capacity (for which dynamic risk factors may be a proxy, see Chap. 2). To illustrate, most people value satisfying interpersonal relationships. It is arguably impossible to promote satisfying prosocial relationships when clients lack the skills required to develop respectful, mutually satisfying adult relationships and/or have high levels of emotional identification with children. Accordingly, interventions designed to strengthen emotional connections with adults would be an important component of a client's therapy plan by strengthening capacity to attain a PHG and addressing risk-relevant propensities. In this way, the GLM satisfies the RNR need principle. The GLM also accommodates the RNR principles of risk and responsivity. For example, individuals assessed with above average risk for recidivism typically experience greater problems with internal and external capacity to realize PHGs in prosocial ways compared to persons assessed in lower risk categories; therefore, they require greater levels of therapeutic intervention. Individuals assessed with a below average risk for recidivism typically require minimal or no therapeutic intervention and might reap greater benefits through practical support (e.g., provided by a case manager, probation officer, or support network), which ensures external conditions are in place to implement GL plans effectively. The GLM addresses the responsivity principle through its central focus on fulfillment of goods that are prioritized by individual clients and its underpinning in universal human rights and human dignity. Interventions are delivered in ways that highlight and maximize their relevance to the individual. Accordingly, any program that correctly implements the GLM should be at least as effective as programs demonstrating fidelity to the core RNR principles.

Exploring the effectiveness of GLM-derived interventions requires a nuanced approach. It is important to stress that the GLM is a practice framework intended to supply practitioners with an overview of the aims and values underpinning practice, rather than a specific treatment model (Ward & Durrant, 2021; Ward & Maruna, 2007). In essence, it functions as a broad map that needs to be supplemented by specific theories concerning concrete interventions (e.g., cognitive behavioral therapy, dialectical behavior therapy). Research exploring the effectiveness of programs influenced by the GLM can basically be classified into those that use the GLM as a broad map informing intervention (as intended and illustrated throughout this book) and those that have integrated GLM-consistent ideas (e.g., approach-oriented therapy goals, attention to well-being as well as risk reduction), without using the GLM as a framework for intervention. The following sections review empirical research that has examined the effectiveness of integrating GLM concepts into correctional rehabilitation, and review empirical research reporting nascent findings from programs/interventions that have explicitly integrated the GLM as an overarching framework. It should be noted that separating studies reporting outcomes of programs integrating GLM concepts versus those derived from the GLM is rather arbitrary based on how programs are described in journal articles rather than on a specific review of program processes, content, and delivery.

9.3.1 Empirical Research Investigating the Integration of GLM-Related Concepts

Several studies have examined the utility of integrating GLM-related concepts or ideas into correctional rehabilitation programs. In one of the first such studies, Mann et al. (2004) compared a traditional, avoidant-goal-focused relapse prevention intervention (e.g., including identifying high risk situations and outlining ways to avoid such situations) with an adapted approach-goal focused intervention. The approach-goal focused intervention used Haaven et al.'s (1990) new me/old me strategy, wherein clients developed approach-oriented goals focused on achieving their "new me" conceptualization, similar to a good lives conceptualization. Forty-seven individuals with convictions for sexual offenses were randomly assigned to the approach-goal or avoidant-goal intervention. Results indicated that participants in the approach-goal oriented intervention engaged better in treatment (as measured by between-session task completion and participants' willingness to disclose problem areas) and were more genuinely motivated to live an offense-free life after treatment (as rated by therapists) compared to participants in the avoidant-goal oriented intervention. Both groups demonstrated similar pre/post-treatment improvements in relapse prevention knowledge and on a measure of self-esteem.

Ware and Bright (2008) reported preliminary findings following changes made to a prison-based sexual offense-focused treatment program in response to a high attrition rate. These changes included switching from closed to open/rolling groups, greater use of approach (versus avoidant) goals, greater emphasis on positive therapist characteristics, and "structuring treatment to reflect the good lives model" (p. 347), with a dual focus on promoting client goals alongside management of recidivism risk. In the absence of formal evaluation data, Ware and Bright reported on short-term observations following program changes, which included a reduced attrition rate, staff feeling more effective and positive in their work (likely benefiting their therapeutic relationship, itself related to treatment change; e.g., Marshall et al., 2003; Serran et al., 2003), and clients exercising greater autonomy in the rehabilitation process through working toward therapy foci at their own pace. For example, high functioning and highly motivated clients were able to complete the program in a shorter time period (6 months) than they could previously (8–10 months).

The GLM's focus on goods fulfillment necessitates a much broader focus than typical correctional rehabilitation programs. In addition to addressing internal capacity for change, external resources and opportunities require consideration. Finding employment represents a common reentry concern. Depending on the individual, employment might help satisfy several PHGs, including mastery in work, agency, states of happiness and pleasure, and creativity. Using a quasi-experimental design, Martin et al. (2010) investigated whether inclusion of an intervention directly assisting clients to find and maintain employment was more effective than social cognitive training (a program targeting criminogenic needs) alone. Their sample comprised 117 individuals, mostly convicted for repeat property and/or drug offenses. A social worker facilitated the employment intervention, which involved securing jobs through liaising with external agencies and assisting participants to retain their jobs. The authors reported no significant between-group differences based on age, educational level, type of offense, sentence duration, and stages of correctional classification. After a 6-year follow-up, survival analyses showed that the social cognitive skills program produced a statistically significant delay in time to reoffense compared to a control group made up of individuals eligible to receive either intervention but did not (for reasons not described by Martin et al.). Although not significant (perhaps due to low statistical power—only 12 participants received the employment intervention), participants receiving both social cognitive training and the employment intervention displayed a longer time to reoffense (and lower percentage of reoffenses) than participants receiving social cognitive training alone. Thus, the employment intervention may have strengthened the effects of the social cognitive training program. As suggested by Martin et al., preparing participants to get and keep a job might increase motivation to engage in rehabilitation programs, thereby indirectly contributing to reductions in recidivism.

Marshall et al.'s (2011) Rockwood program for sexual offending incorporates many GLM-related concepts, including approach-oriented treatment goals and a modified version of the GLM. This is introduced early in their program and used toward the end to integrate learning from previous phases and prepare clients for discharge. Marshall et al. stated that "the final phase of the program aims at integrating what has been learned so far into plans for release and for the continued development of a more fulfilling life. The first step involves identifying the goals and plans to achieve these goals, within the framework of our version of the GLM" (p. 156). In their modified version of the GLM, the PHGs are condensed into six areas: "health (good diet and exercise), mastery (in work and play), autonomy (agency/self-directiveness), relatedness (intimate/sexual relationship, family friends, kinship, and community), inner peace (freedom from turmoil and stress, a sense of purpose and meaning in life), knowledge and creativity (satisfaction from knowing and creating things—job—or hobby-related knowledge, playing music, writing)" (Exhibit 7.2, p. 127). An evaluation of an early version of Rockwood's program ($n = 579$) compared recidivism outcomes with the Correctional Service of Canada's (CSC) standard sexual offense treatment program (CBT/RNR; $n = 625$) and an untreated comparison group ($n = 107$) (Olver et al., 2020). Rates of sexual reoffending after an 8-year fixed follow-up period were lower for both treatment groups (4.2% and 10.7% for Rockwood and CSC, respectively) compared to the comparison group (20.2%), with the Rockwood program demonstrating the lowest recidivism rates overall. Olver et al.'s findings provide some of the strongest evidence to date for the added effectiveness of strengths-based approaches over and above risk/deficit-based approaches to correctional rehabilitation.

Thus far, we have reviewed a selection of empirical studies describing interventions that have incorporated GLM-related concepts, including the use of approach-oriented treatment goals and extending the focus of interventions to attend to client well-being alongside the traditional emphasis on risk reduction. Findings are encouraging, suggesting the addition of strengths-based elements helps to address key problems evident with a narrow risk management approach. The following section considers those studies that have reported findings from interventions that have explicitly integrated the GLM as an overarching practice framework.

9.3.2 Empirical Research Investigating GLM-Derived Interventions

This book describes and illustrates what constitutes GLM-derived interventions. Yet programs described as "GLM-informed" vary in the extent to which the GLM informs various aspects of intervention. Across a multisite study exploring the application of the GLM in 13 North American sexual offending treatment programs, operationalization of the GLM included reframing program components using approach versus avoidant goals, adopting a stronger individualized rather than one-size-fits all approach through individualized treatment/intervention plans, adopting a holistic focus beyond criminogenic needs, and engaging with clients with dignity and respect as fellow human beings (Willis et al., 2014). All these strategies are consistent with a GLM approach; however, on their own, they fall short of what might be considered a GLM-derived intervention. The GLM was largely absent from assessment practices and protocols, and individualized intervention plans often amounted to extra space for client goals to be added to generic treatment goals. Most programs were considered to show some responsiveness to the GLM; however, GLM application was largely additive to a dominating risk management or relapse prevention (RP) framework. It is therefore prudent when reviewing evaluations of interventions claiming to use the GLM that we ask whether the intervention is indeed derived from the GLM, or if it is better described as integrating GLM-related concepts.

In this chapter, separation of studies integrating GLM concepts versus those derived from the GLM was somewhat arbitrary and based on available publications. However, the approach here was consistent with criteria put forward in two recent systematic reviews examining the effectiveness of GLM-derived interventions (Mallion et al., 2020; Zeccola et al., 2021). Mallion et al.'s criteria for a GLM-consistent program included: assessment of the client's valued PHGs, identification of obstacles to goods attainment through prosocial means, development of a GLP, and use of the GLP to guide intervention. Zeccola et al.'s criteria were similar, namely, explicit incorporation of risk reduction and well-being enhancement, assessment of PHGs, and individualized intervention plans centered on attainment of PHGs. Mallion et al. included studies reporting varied outcomes (recidivism, pre/post-treatment changes, and service user perspectives; note that case studies were excluded) and identified five studies meeting their criteria (Barnett et al., 2014; Harkins et al., 2012; Leeson & Adshead, 2013; Mann et al., 2004; Ward & Attwell, 2014). Zeccola et al.'s review was restricted to studies reporting on recidivism outcomes or pre/post-treatment changes to dynamic risk factors (DRFs), including case studies; six studies met their criteria (Barnett et al., 2014; Gannon et al., 2011; Harkins et al., 2012; Lindsay et al., 2007; Whitehead et al., 2007; Wylie & Griffin, 2013). The majority of studies included across both reviews focused on adult samples, with two exceptions (Leeson & Adshead, 2013; Wylie & Griffin, 2013). Mallion et al.'s (2020) findings suggested that GLM-derived interventions were equally effective to standard RP interventions based on pre/post-treatment psychometric change to variables aligning with DRFs. Additionally, they found that GLM-derived interventions were associated with improved treatment motivation and engagement along with positive service user perspectives. No studies in their review reported on recidivism outcomes. Zeccola et al.'s (2021) systematic review reported on two of the same pre/post-treatment change studies as Mallion et al. (Barnett et al., 2014; Harkins et al., 2012) and the remaining four papers utilized case study or case series designs. They concluded that there was insufficient evidence to ascertain whether GLM-derived interventions were associated with reductions in actual recidivism. However, there was some evidence that GLM-derived interventions appeared effective at reducing recidivism risk and no indications that the GLM was associated with increased recidivism risk.

Two studies reporting on pre/post-treatment change were included in both Mallion et al.'s (2020) and Zeccola et al.'s (2021) systematic reviews (Barnett et al., 2014; Harkins et al., 2012). Harkins et al. (2012) conducted an evaluation of the better lives module, introduced as a replacement to an RP-oriented module for individuals convicted of sexual offenses and living in the community in the United Kingdom. The better lives module was developed using a GLM approach and involved promoting prosocial attainment of each of the GLM primary goods. Several comparisons were made between clients who participated in the RP-oriented module ($n = 701$) and the better lives module ($n = 76$). Although there were no differences in attrition rates or treatment change (as measured using a psychometric battery), both facilitators and program participants described the better lives module more positively. Of note, most of the facilitators interviewed reported that the better lives module did not pay sufficient (if any) attention to criminogenic needs. Accordingly, the program was amended to better reflect the GLM's twin focus of risk reduction and well-being enhancement. Barnett et al. (2014) evaluated the amended program, comparing changes in psychometric scores for individuals who had participated in the amended program versus the traditional RP program ($N = 601$). They found little difference in change on psychometric measures (including measures of risk, empathy, recognition of lapse cues, self-esteem, loneliness, attitudes toward the sexual abuse of children, assertiveness, and locus of control) between the two groups and no difference in attrition rates. A greater proportion of the participants in the GLM program attained a "treated profile" (i.e., one that was indistinguishable from a group of people who had not offended) than in the RP group; however, this finding did not account for pretreatment scores for the RP group that were more dysfunctional than the GLM group. The authors emphasized that further research was required to understand differences between RP and GLM-derived treatment programs.

Across diverse case studies included in Zeccola et al.'s review, findings supported the premise that strengthening client capacity to achieve primary goods in prosocial ways may promote desistance from offending. For example, Whitehead et al. (2007) applied the GLM with an individual who was convicted for violent offenses and assessed at high risk for reoffending. Whitehead et al. reported that the implementation of GLM principles facilitated treatment readiness, and promoted long-term reintegration goals, including engaging in university study and developing prosocial leisure pursuits. Both activities encouraged moving away from associating with an antisocial peer group (itself a DRF for violent recidivism; Bonta & Andrews, 2024) and increased association with a prosocial peer group. Official statistics revealed that the individual concerned was not convicted of a new crime after approximately 6 years.

At least one study evaluated outcomes of a GLM-informed intervention that was not included in Mallion et al.'s (2020) or Zeccola et al.'s (2021) systematic reviews likely because "GLM" was not included in the article title or keywords, and therefore not identified by the search strategy of either review. Tyler et al. (2018) evaluated a specialty treatment program for persons residing in forensic psychiatric hospitals with a history of deliberate fire setting ($N = 63$). The GLM was introduced early in the program and integrated throughout session content, with the program culminating in development of a future-oriented good lives plan. Compared to a treatment-as-usual comparison group, participants demonstrated significant pre/post-treatment change on fire-related measures and anger expression, as measured with a psychometric battery. Participants were additionally asked to rate their satisfaction with treatment, including rating how important they viewed each aspect of the program to their individual progress. "Learning about good lives and how to create a more satisfying life for myself" (p. 397) was one of the most important aspects of treatment as rated by consumers, alongside fire-related psychoeducational components.

Taken together, research reviewed in this chapter suggests that the GLM offers a more engaging rehabilitation approach compared to more traditional risk/deficit-based approaches. However, two recent systematic reviews identified just nine distinct studies evaluating what were considered GLM-derived interventions. Nascent research is encouraging, but at the same time illuminates the difficulties inherent in evaluating GLM-derived interventions. That the GLM is not a prescribed treatment program readily amenable to evaluation is both a strength and a challenge. The challenge is that it makes evaluation more difficult (than, e.g., dichotomous ratings of adherence to each of the Risk, Need, & Responsivity principles; e.g., Hanson et al., 2009), but its strength is its alignment with what we know from general psychotherapy literature about how individuals change (see Wampold & Imel, 2015). Next are some implications for advancing empirical research into GLM-derived interventions.

9.4 Implications for Future Research

The GLM faces numerous challenges to implementation—and therefore evaluation—which will be expanded on with policy implications in Chap. 10. Briefly, the ethical values at the core of the GLM emphasizing universal human rights are difficult to uphold in sociopolitical environments that favor retributive approaches to justice over restorative, humanistic approaches. Relatedly, fiscal pressures have contributed to a growing reliance on paraprofessionals to deliver structured, manualized, offense-focused programs (Forde, 2017; Gannon & Ward, 2014), which is inconsistent with the flexible, collaborative therapeutic approach advocated by the GLM. Thus, there is a paucity of empirical research supporting the GLM and calls for more research, even as the sociopolitical environment in which correctional rehabilitation is embedded constrains implementation of the GLM. Advancing empirical research thus requires engaging all key stakeholders, as research evaluating GLM-derived interventions necessitates environments that support their existence.

As previously highlighted, substantial variation exists in how the GLM has been operationalized in practice (e.g., Willis et al., 2014). Future research might benefit from a metric that assesses the extent to which the GLM practice framework informs all aspects of an intervention, such that those demonstrating greater adherence to the GLM can be evaluated against those with weaker adherence. Such a metric might be informed by existing guidelines for integrating the GLM across correctional rehabilitation programs (see Willis et al., 2013), and the GLM fidelity monitoring tool introduced in Chap. 4 (Prescott et al., 2024).

It may be worth broadening the range of outcome measures used as indicators of intervention effectiveness. Outcome measures in extant research are often limited to officially recorded recidivism and pre/post-treatment psychometric change to variables mapping onto DRFs. Notwithstanding questionable reliability and validity of some of the psychometrics used in extant research (see Grady et al., 2011), as highlighted in Chap. 2, there are several conceptual problems with DRFs that undermine their legitimacy as causal factors for offending, and by extension, as intervention targets. Furthermore, measuring change to risk-related variables to evaluate therapy effectiveness is inconsistent with the holistic focus of the GLM. Given its dual focus on preventing future offending and assisting clients to live more fulfilling, meaningful lives, an important implication for future research is developing outcome measures that focus on the extent to which therapy clients can pursue PHGs in adaptive, prosocial, and meaningful ways. Olson et al.'s (2024) GLAD scale represents a promising advancement in this direction. Olson et al.'s study offers the first validated scale to assess attainment of PHGs and accordingly offers researchers a new means for assessing intervention outcomes beyond simple consideration of reoffending outcomes. Without tracking change in clients' pursuit of PHGs, the effectiveness of GLM-derived interventions will remain somewhat concealed. Simply put, an absence of recidivism does not equate to effective implementation of a GLP, realization of good life goals, or desistance from future offending. Given that living in line with a GLP is incompatible with offending, analysis of GLM-specific outcomes might provide a more sensitive indicator of intervention effectiveness than recidivism data alone.

Alongside further development and validation of GLM-specific measures, future research might examine pre/post-intervention changes to protective factors. Protective factors reflect the presence of prosocial attributes associated with reductions in reoffending (de Vogel et al., 2012; de Vries Robbé et al., 2015), and evidence for the validity of clinician-rated measures of protective factors is accumulating (Burghart et al., 2023; Thornton et al., 2024; Wanamaker et al., 2018). As discussed in Chap. 3, within the GLM practice framework, protective factors represent proxies for strengths in an individual's capacity to implement a prosocial GLP, and their assessment better aligns with the GLM than an assessment of DRFs. Moreover, a recent study applying a network approach to understanding dynamic risk and protective factors with 317 forensic psychiatric patients found that protective factors were more central (considering individual item associations with all risk and protective factors assessed) than risk factors (Bogaerts et al., 2020). The authors concluded that their findings supported interventions focused on building strengths and competencies and thus aligned well with the GLM. Accordingly, at a time when sociopolitical environments make implementing GLM-derived interventions challenging, clinicians and researchers might consider broadening the range of outcome measures selected to evaluate intervention effectiveness. Finally, expanding the focus of empirical research beyond offense-focused treatment to external capacity/environmental considerations (e.g., access to employment and other prosocial means for securing PHGs) will also advance the GLM's evidence base. Findings from such studies might generate the data necessary to build a stronger case for GLM-informed correctional interventions than what is available at the time of publication of this book.

9.5 Conclusion

There is burgeoning evidence supporting the knowledge-related assumptions of the GLM, and those interventions derived from them. With a new generation of GLM-aligned, strengths-based outcome measures in various stages of development and validation, hopefully empirical research will continue to accumulate in the coming years. In the meantime, the GLM is well established in forensic/correctional psychology practice and offers a strengths-based rehabilitation framework that aligns with the extensively researched RNR principles. Despite challenges to its empirical evaluation, the GLM aligns well with the rich and impressive criminological literature on desistance from crime (e.g., Laub & Sampson, 2003). According to researchers such as Porporino (2010) and Laws and Ward (2011), desistance research underlines the necessity of incorporating community-based factors such as employment or education within rehabilitation programs. However, it is never going to be enough to simply assign someone a job or enroll them in an educational program and hope that they will succeed. The GLM is ideally placed to reinforce desistance processes through its sensitivity to an individual's core commitments, practical identities, and social ecology. It supports clients and clinicians in identifying those opportunities with maximum potential to act as turning points, and provides a systematic, comprehensive framework for intervention and ongoing case management to capitalize on such opportunities. Simply addressing risk factors is unlikely to encourage individuals who have committed crimes to adopt socially adaptive and personally meaningful ways of thinking about themselves and others. We hope this chapter offers inspiration to the next generation of researchers to further the evidence base for the GLM, and in doing so, promote more humane, engaging, and ultimately effective approaches to working with people who have caused harm.

References

Andrews, D. A., Bonta, J., & Wormith, J. S. (2011). The Risk-Need-Responsivity (RNR) Model: Does adding the Good Lives Model contribute to effective crime prevention? *Criminal Justice and Behavior, 38*, 735–755. https://doi.org/10.1177/0093854811406356

Appiah, O. K., & Billen, E. (2024). Evaluating the Good Lives Model among students: The role of primary goods and self-regulation in achieving a good life. *Journal of Forensic Psychology Research and Practice*, 1–27. https://doi.org/10.1080/24732850.2024.2394528

Barendregt, C. S. (2015). *Needs, risks, and protective factors of adolescents in secure residential care: Identification of a conceptual model based on the Good Lives Model* [Tilburg University]. Ipskamp Drukkers. https://pure.uvt.nl/ws/portalfiles/portal/25642852/Barendregt_Needs_06_03_2015_emb_tot_01_05_2018_aangep_Dankwoord_eruit.pdf

Barendregt, C. S., Van der Laan, A. M., Bongers, I. L., & Van Nieuwenhuizen, C. (2018). Quality of life, delinquency and psychosocial functioning of adolescents in secure residential care: Testing two assumptions of the Good Lives Model. *Child and Adolescent Psychiatry and Mental Health, 12*, Article 4. https://doi.org/10.1186/s13034-017-0209-9

Barnett, G. D., Manderville-Norden, R., & Rakestrow, J. (2014). The Good Lives Model or relapse prevention: What works better in facilitating change? *Sexual Abuse, 26*(1), 3–33. https://doi.org/10.1177/1079063212474473

Bogaerts, S., Spreen, M., Masthoff, E., & Jankovic, M. (2020). Longitudinal network structure and changes of clinical risk and protective factors in a nationwide sample of forensic psychiatric patients. *International Journal of Offender Therapy and Comparative Criminology, 64*(15), 1533–1550. https://doi.org/10.1177/0306624x20923256

Bonta, J., & Andrews, D. A. (2003). A commentary on Ward and Stewart's model of human needs. *Psychology, Crime and Law, 9*, 215–218. https://doi.org/10.1080/10683/16031000112115

Bonta, J., & Andrews, D. A. (2024). *The psychology of criminal conduct* (7th ed.). Routledge.

Burghart, M., de Ruiter, C., Hynes, S. E., Krishnan, N., Levtova, Y., & Uyar, A. (2023). The Structured Assessment of Protective Factors for violence risk (SAPROF): A meta-analysis of its predictive and incremental validity. *Psychological Assessment, 35*(1), 56–67. https://doi.org/10.1037/pas0001184

Chu, C. M., Koh, L. L., Zeng, G., & Teoh, J. (2015). Youth who sexually offended: Primary human goods and offense pathways. *Sexual Abuse, 27*, 151–172. https://doi.org/10.1177/1079063213499188

de Vogel, V., de Ruiter, C., Bouman, Y., & de Vries Robbé, M. (2012). *SAPROF. Guidelines for the assessment of protective factors for violence risk* (2nd ed.). Van der Hoeven Stichting.

de Vries Robbé, M., Mann, R. E., Maruna, S., & Thornton, D. (2015). An exploration of protective factors supporting desistance from sexual offending. *Sexual Abuse, 27*(1), 16–33. https://doi.org/10.1177/1079063214547582

Fazel, S., Hurton, C., Burghart, M., DeLisi, M., & Yu, R. (2024). An updated evidence synthesis on the Risk-Need-Responsivity (RNR) model: Umbrella review and commentary. *Journal of Criminal Justice, 92*, 102197. https://doi.org/10.1016/j.jcrimjus.2024.102197

Forde, R. A. (2017). *Bad psychology: How forensic psychology left science behind*. Jessica Kingsley Publishers.

Gannon, T. A., King, T., Miles, H., Lockerbie, L., & Willis, G. M. (2011). Good lives sexual offender treatment for mentally disordered offenders. *British Journal of Forensic Practice, 13*(3), 153–168. https://doi.org/10.1108/14636641111157805

Gannon, T. A., Olver, M. E., Mallion, J. S., & James, M. (2019). Does specialized psychological treatment for offending reduce recidivism? A meta-analysis examining staff and program variables as predictors of treatment effectiveness. *Clinical Psychology Review, 73*, 101752. https://doi.org/10.1016/j.cpr.2019.101752

Gannon, T. A., & Ward, T. (2014). Where has all the psychology gone? A critical review of evidence-based psychological practice in correctional settings. *Aggression and Violent Behavior, 19*, 435–446. https://doi.org/10.1016/j.avb.2014.06.006

Grady, M. D., Brodersen, M., & Abramson, J. M. (2011). The state of psychological measures for adult sexual offenders. *Aggression and Violent Behavior, 16*, 227–240. https://doi.org/10.1016/j.avb.2011.03.001

Haaven, J., Little, R., & Petre-Miller, D. (1990). *Treating intellectually disabled sex offenders: A model residential program*. Safer Society Press.

Hanson, R. K., Bourgon, G., Helmus, L., & Hodgson, S. (2009). The principles of effective correctional treatment also apply to sexual offenders: A meta-analysis. *Criminal Justice and Behavior, 36*, 865–891. https://doi.org/10.1177/0093854809338545

Harkins, L., Flak, V. E., Beech, A., & Woodhams, J. (2012). Evaluation of a community-based sex offender treatment program using a Good Lives Model approach. *Sexual Abuse, 24*(6), 519–543. https://doi.org/10.1177/1079063211429469

Laub, J. H., & Sampson, R. J. (2003). *Shared beginnings, divergent lives: Delinquent boys to age 70*. Harvard University Press.

Laws, D. R., & Ward, T. (2011). *Desistance from sex offending: Alternatives to throwing away the keys*. Guilford Press.

Leeson, S., & Adshead, M. (2013). The response of adolescents and practitioners to a Good Lives approach. In B. Print & T. Ward (Eds.), *The Good Lives Model for adolescents who sexually harm* (pp. 183–193). Safer Society Press.

Lindsay, W. R., Ward, T., Morgan, T., & Wilson, I. (2007). Self-regulation of sex offending, future pathways and the Good Lives Model: Applications and problems. *Journal of Sexual Aggression, 13*, 37–50. https://doi.org/10.1080/13552600701365613

Loney, D. M., & Harkins, L. (2018). Examining the good lives model and antisocial behaviour. *Psychology, Crime & Law, 24*(1), 38–51. https://doi.org/10.1080/1068316X.2017.1371304

Mallion, J. S. (2021). *Application of the Good Lives Model to street gang members*. University of Kent.

Mallion, J. S., Wood, J. L., & Mallion, A. (2020). Systematic review of 'Good Lives' assumptions and interventions. *Aggression and Violent Behavior, 55*, 101510. https://doi.org/10.1016/j.avb.2020.101510

Mann, R. E. (2000). Managing resistance and rebellion in relapse prevention intervention. In D. R. Laws, S. M. Hudson, & T. Ward (Eds.), *Remaking relapse prevention with sex offenders: A sourcebook* (pp. 187–200). Sage Publications.

Mann, R. E., Webster, S. D., Schofield, C., & Marshall, W. L. (2004). Approach versus avoidance goals in relapse prevention with sexual offenders. *Sexual Abuse, 16*(1), 65–75. https://doi.org/10.1177/107906320401600105

Marshall, W. L., Marshall, L. E., Serran, G. A., & O'Brien, M. D. (2011). *Rehabilitating sexual offenders: A strength-based approach*. American Psychological Association.

Marshall, W. L., Serran, G. A., Fernandez, Y. M., Mulloy, R., Mann, R. E., & Thornton, D. (2003). Therapist characteristics in the treatment of sexual offenders: Tentative data on their relationship with indices of behaviour change. *Journal of Sexual Aggression, 9*, 25–30. https://doi.org/10.1080/355260031000137940

Martin, A. M., Hernandez, B., Hernandez-Fernaud, E., Arregui, J. L., & Hernandez, J. A. (2010). The enhancement effect of social and employment integration on the delay of recidivism of released offenders trained with the R & R programme. *Psychology, Crime & Law, 16*, 401–413. https://doi.org/10.1080/10683160902776835

Norcross, J. C. (2002). *Psychotherapy relationships that work: Therapist contributions and responsiveness to patients* (3rd ed.). Oxford University Press. https://doi.org/10.1093/med-psych/9780190843953.001.0001

Olson, J., Giever, D., & Sarver, R. S. (2024). Validation of the good lives assessment of domains in an adult US sample. *International Journal of Offender Therapy and Comparative Criminology*. Advance online publication. https://doi.org/10.1177/0306624X241240711

Olver, M. E., Marshall, L. E., Marshall, W. L., & Nicholaichuk, T. P. (2020). A long-term outcome assessment of the effects on subsequent reoffense rates of a prison-based CBT/RNR sex offender treatment program with strength-based elements. *Sexual Abuse, 32*, 127–153. https://doi.org/10.1177/1079063218807486

Porporino, F. J. (2010). Bringing sense and sensitivity to corrections: From programmes to 'fix' offenders to services to support desistance. In J. Brayford, F. Cowe, & J. Deering (Eds.), *What else works? Creative work with offenders*. Willan Publishing.

Prescott, D. S., Willis, G. M., & Ward, T. (2024). Monitoring therapist fidelity to the Good Lives Model (GLM). *International Journal of Offender Therapy and Comparative Criminology, 68*(1). https://doi.org/10.1177/0306624X221086572

Purvis, M. (2005). *Seeking a good life: Human goods and sexual offending*. University of Melbourne.

Purvis, M. (2010). *Seeking a good life: Human Goods and Sexual Offending*. Lambert Academic Press.

Serran, G., Fernandez, Y., Marshall, W. L., & Mann, R. E. (2003). Process issues in treatment: Application to sexual offender programs. *Professional Psychology: Research and Practice, 34*, 368–374.

Taylor, E. (2017). 'I should have been a security consultant': The Good Lives Model and residential burglars. *European Journal of Criminology, 14*, 434–450. https://doi.org/10.1177/1477370816661743

Thornton, D., Willis, G. M., & Kelley, S. (2024). Dynamic protective factors relevant to sexual offending. *Current Psychiatry Reports*. https://doi.org/10.1007/s11920-024-01493-5

Tyler, N., Gannon, T. A., Lockerbie, L., Ciardha, Ó., & C. (2018). An evaluation of a specialist firesetting treatment programme for male and female mentally disordered offenders (the FIP-MO). *Clinical Psychology & Psychotherapy, 25*, 388–400. https://doi.org/10.1002/cpp.2172

Van Damme, L., Hoeve, M., Vermeiren, R., Vanderplasschen, W., & Colins, O. F. (2016). Quality of life in relation to future mental health problems and offending: Testing the good lives model among detained girls. *Law and Human Behavior, 40*(3), 285–294. https://doi.org/10.1037/lhb0000177

Wampold, B. E., & Imel, Z. E. (2015). *The great psychotherapy debate: Models, methods, and findings* (2nd ed.). Routledge.

Wanamaker, K. A., Jones, N. J., & Brown, S. L. (2018). Strengths-based assessments for use with forensic populations: A critical review. *International Journal of Forensic Mental Health, 17*(2), 202–221. https://doi.org/10.1080/14999013.2018.1451414

Ward, M., & Attwell, P. (2014). Evaluation of two community outreach forensic psychological services. *Journal of Forensic Practice, 16*, 312–326. https://doi.org/10.1108/JFP-04-2013-0027

Ward, T., & Durrant, R. (2021). Practice frameworks in correctional psychology: Translating causal theories and normative assumptions into practice. *Aggression and Violent Behavior, 58*, 101612. https://doi.org/10.1016/j.avb.2021.101612

Ward, T., & Maruna, S. (2007). *Rehabilitation: Beyond the risk assessment paradigm*. Routledge.

Ward, T., Yates, P. M., & Willis, G. M. (2012). The Good Lives Model and the risk need responsivity model: A critical response to Andrews, Bonta, and Wormith (2011). *Criminal Justice and Behavior, 39*, 94–110. https://doi.org/10.1177/0093854811426085

Ware, J., & Bright, D. A. (2008). Evolution of a treatment programme for sex offenders: Changes to the NSW Custody-Based Intensive Treatment (CUBIT). *Psychiatry, Psychology and Law, 15*, 340–349. https://doi.org/10.1080/13218710802014543

Whitehead, P. R., Ward, T., & Collie, R. M. (2007). Time for a change: Applying the Good Lives Model of rehabilitation to a high-risk violent offender. *International Journal of Offender Therapy and Comparative Criminology, 51*(5), 578–598. https://doi.org/10.1177/0306624X06296236

Willis, G. M., & Grace, R. C. (2008). The quality of community reintegration planning for child molesters: Effects on sexual recidivism. *Sexual Abuse, 20*, 218–240. https://doi.org/10.1177/1079063208318005

Willis, G. M., & Ward, T. (2011). Striving for a good life: The Good Lives Model applied to released child molesters. *Journal of Sexual Aggression, 17*, 290–303. https://doi.org/10.1080/13552600.2010.505349

Willis, G. M., & Ward, T. (2024). Evidence for the Good Lives Model in supporting rehabilitation and desistance from offending. In L. Craig, L. Dixon, & T. A. Gannon (Eds.), *The Wiley handbook of what works in correctional rehabilitation: An evidence-based approach to theory, assessment and treatment* (2nd ed.). Wiley.

Willis, G. M., Ward, T., & Levenson, J. S. (2014). The Good Lives Model (GLM): An evaluation of GLM operationalization in North American treatment programs. *Sexual Abuse, 26*, 58–81. https://doi.org/10.1177/1079063213478202

Willis, G. M., Yates, P. M., Gannon, T. A., & Ward, T. (2013). How to integrate the Good Lives Model into treatment programs for sexual offending: An introduction and overview. *Sexual Abuse, 25*, 123–142. https://doi.org/10.1177/1079063212452618

Wormith, J. S., Gendreau, P., & Bonta, J. (2012). Deferring to clarity, parsimony, and evidence in reply to Ward, Yates, and Willis. *Criminal Justice and Behavior, 39*, 111–120. https://doi.org/10.1177/0093854811426087

Wylie, L. A., & Griffin, H. L. (2013). G-map's application of the Good Lives Model to adolescent males who sexually harm: A case study. *Journal of Sexual Aggression, 19*(3), 345–356. https://doi.org/10.1080/13552600.2011.650715

Yates, P. M. (2009). Using the Good Lives Model to motivate sexual offenders to participate in treatment. In D. S. Prescott (Ed.), *Building motivation to change in sexual offenders* (pp. 74–95). Safer Society Press.

Zeccola, J., Kelty, S. F., & Boer, D. (2021). Does the good lives model work? A systematic review of the recidivism evidence. *The Journal of Forensic Practice, 23*(3), 285–300. https://doi.org/10.1108/JFP-03-2021-0010

Chapter 10
Policy Implications

10.1 Introduction

The chapters of this book have described and illustrated how the good lives model (GLM) informs strengths-based correctional interventions, with the overall aim of equipping practitioners with the knowledge and clinical resources necessary to implement the GLM across forensic/correctional settings. Yet correctional interventions don't exist within a vacuum. Effective operationalization of the GLM requires not only skilled clinicians, but environments that afford clients opportunities to implement a good life plan. In their evaluation of GLM operationalization across 13 North American sexual offending treatment programs, Willis et al. (2014) found that the biggest barriers hindering GLM implementation related to policy and legislation, including probation/parole conditions alongside contemporary sex crime legislation such as residence restrictions. This chapter[1] will focus on the broad policy implications of the GLM, starting with a brief review of the GLM practice framework and highlighting some key considerations in relation to correctional policy. Next is an examination of policy implications for rehabilitation in institutional settings, including descriptions of the development and some key characteristics of a recent alternative to traditional prisons (i.e., detention houses) and their alignment with the GLM, with the situation in Belgium used as a case example. We then discuss community-based policy implications, analyzing contemporary policy for its alignment with the GLM, with a focus on sex crime policies given their widespread implementation and implications. We conclude with some reflections on broader justice system-level implications of the GLM.

[1] We would like to sincerely thank Petra Colpaert, manager, and Daisy Steen, former psychologist, of the detention house in Kortrijk, for their valuable comments, ideas, and suggestions.

T. Ward et al., *The Good Lives Model of Correctional Rehabilitation*,
Advances in Preventing and Treating Violence and Aggression,
https://doi.org/10.1007/978-3-031-95559-4_10

10.2 The Good Lives Model Practice Framework Applied to Correctional Policy

At its core, the GLM supports human agency, self-determination, and self-regulation. It was introduced to address key limitations of the risk-need-responsivity (RNR) model of correctional rehabilitation (Bonta & Andrews, 2017), expanding the focus of rehabilitation to consider client well-being alongside risk reduction. A key etiological assumption of the GLM is that antisocial/criminal behavior is characterized by impairments in individuals' good lives plans, including problematic ways of seeking primary goods. Essentially, the GLM offers insight into why people commit crimes and the function of offending behavior with respect to an individual's core commitments and priorities in life. Using the GLM, rehabilitation aims to support clients' pursuit of primary human goods (PHGs) in personally meaningful ways that do not result in harm to members of the community and to society more generally.

The GLM emphasizes the ethical values of universal human rights, human dignity, and human agency. Thus, correctional policies that unduly undermine human rights, disrespect human dignity, and/or restrict one's agency beyond what is ethically justified to ensure that the rights of other people are respected risk undermining an individual's capacity to implement a good life plan (Ward & Salmon, 2009). On the surface, criminal justice sanctions clearly impede an individual's agency by curtailing their freedom of movement and access to certain services and goods; however, sanctions can be delivered in ways that uphold human rights and minimally constrain agency (Ward & Birgden, 2007). Numerous contemporary correctional policies undermine the GLM practice framework, including (and certainly not limited to) denying individuals in prison the right to vote, restricting or prohibiting contact with social supports, and forced castration. Essentially, any policy that removes adaptive, prosocial access to one or more primary goods without a sound ethical or safety justification can undermine the implementation of the GLM.

More broadly, language used across correctional systems can align with or undermine GLM-grounded rehabilitation and reintegration. Language consistent with the GLM recognizes that individuals who have committed crimes are "people like us." For example, when housed in institutions, they might be referred to as "residents." Referring to them as "offenders," by their surname only, or by a number is not consistent with underlying ethical values of the GLM, which insist on treating all individuals with respect. Similarly, policies that label a person based on a criminal conviction (e.g., a "sex offender," "child molester," or "fire-setter") are also inconsistent with the GLM, of which there are several. For example, in the USA and elsewhere, most persons convicted for sexual offenses will be required to register as a "registered sex offender" for many years if not life, with their personal details readily accessible via publicly accessible online registries (Ackerman et al., 2011). Also in the USA, some individuals convicted for sexual offenses are classified as "sexually violent predators" or "SVPs." Research is clear that labeling can increase the risk of future criminality through obstructing prosocial identity change, blocking access to prosocial opportunities, and increasing association with antisocial peers (Chiricos et al., 2007; Restivo & Lanier, 2015). In other words, offense-based labeling seriously infringes on the external capacity required for individuals who have offended to implement a prosocial good life Plan (GLP). Instead, labels categorize and define a person on the basis of past behavior—the very behavior we seek to prevent (e.g., Willis, 2018). Thus, a fundamental consideration when using the GLM is attention to the language used in correctional policy, rehabilitation program names, and more broadly in communication with key stakeholders and the general public. The continued use of labels will undoubtedly contribute to the continued marginalization of individuals who have offended, blocking their access to PHGs in ways that the rest of us take for granted. Instead, the GLM advocates for using respectful language that aligns with an individual's identity and prosocial pursuits. When referring to an individual or groups of people in the justice system, person-first language provides an alternative to offense-based labels. For example, we might refer to individuals/adults/young people previously convicted for sexual (or other) offenses or with a history of sexual (or other) offending. In this way, the person is separated from an offense or past behavior and not defined by it. When referring to an individual or groups with a known prosocial identity, identity-first language can be appropriate. For example, many people with disabilities prefer identity-first language (e.g., Deaf person) over person-first language (e.g., people with hearing loss; Dunn & Andrews, 2015). Similarly, some people attracted to children self-identify as a minor attracted person or MAP (B4U-ACT, 2019). With the ethical value of respecting human dignity at its core, the GLM advocates for using language consistent with people's preferences, and when these are unknown, person-first language offers a more respectful alternative to commonly used derogatory labels.

An organization or government's official policies guide actions and can impact profoundly on individual lives and society. For example, following the outbreak of Covid-19, governments internationally introduced various policies in an attempt to contain its spread, which at the peak of the pandemic, included national lockdowns. Effective policies were critical for alleviating adverse effects on society, including increased mortality rates. Policies included travel restrictions, isolation and quarantine, social distancing, and requirements to wear personal protective equipment (PPE), including face masks. Across a sample of 144 countries, stricter government policies were associated with a reduced number of deaths compared to more relaxed policies (Chisadza et al., 2021). Although there may have been some exceptions, Covid-19 policies made intuitive sense, were informed by research, and ultimately proved effective. Through a GLM lens, although available means to attain primary goods were restricted at the peak of the pandemic with people unable to socialize, work (outside of essential services), or engage in many leisure activities, Covid-19 policies were generally time-limited and driven by the goal of preventing illness and mortality. We turn now to considering correctional policies in institutional and community settings, and the extent to which they align with the GLM.

10.3 Policy Implications for Institutional Settings

Rehabilitation in line with the GLM requires environments that support the prosocial pursuit and acquisition of PHGs. However, many of the ways in which correctional institutions are organized and operate in western criminal justice jurisdictions are inconsistent with the GLM. An example is solitary confinement, which has been in use since the eighteenth century and continues in prisons all over the world (Silverthorn & Zgoba, 2024). A recent systematic review and meta-analysis (Luigi et al., 2020) found that solitary confinement was associated with harmful effects on psychological well-being, which extend beyond those associated with general incarceration. The results from 13 studies, representing a pooled sample of over 380,000 detained people, showed that solitary confinement exacerbated negative psychological impacts, self-injury, and death rates (Luigi et al., 2020). Based on these results, it is hard to imagine how solitary confinement might offer opportunities for people to acquire PHGs such as inner peace, relatedness, or community. Likewise, it is difficult to fathom how solitary confinement might contribute to reducing recidivism risk, which is underpinned by a recent review and meta-analysis indicating that solitary confinement was associated with increased post-release recidivism (Luigi et al., 2022). The studies in the meta-analysis, all from North America and comprising almost 195,000 detained people in total, showed a moderate association between solitary confinement and recidivism in general. Similar associations were found for solitary confinement and violent recidivism, reincarceration, and rearrests. The study also indicated that the risk of recidivism increased if the solitary confinement was more recent and lengthier in time (Luigi et al., 2022).

Encouragingly, recent changes in correctional policy in some jurisdictions align well with the GLM's core values and principles, knowledge-related assumptions, and intervention guidelines. Policies that allow for temporary releases, in many cases when the end of the prison sentence or release on parole approaches, such as the UK's release on temporary license (ROTL), facilitate contact with family and social networks and make it easier for individuals to seek employment and housing opportunities post-release (Mathlin et al., 2024). Accordingly, such policies can help individuals gain access to PHGs, including agency, relatedness, and excellence in work, because detained people can establish or strengthen social bonds and explore possibilities for rebuilding their lives. Results of a meta-analysis indicated that home leave and work release programs were associated with reduced recidivism, and that work release programs also corresponded with higher rates of post-release employment (Cheliotis, 2008).

"Detention houses," are a particular innovation in Europe, developed as an alternative to traditional prisons, whose conceptual and architectural origins date back to the nineteenth century (Jewkes, 2018). A recent literature review indicated clear links between the prison architecture, its climate, and the well-being of prisoners (Engstrom & van Ginneken, 2022). In this study, the authors refer to several elements of a prison environment that may positively or negatively influence the well-being of people living in correctional settings. These elements include aspects related to one's personal living space (e.g., lighting, noise, temperature, air quality, and privacy) and general prison spaces (e.g., size, prison layout, age of the prison, and availability of services). Based on the review, the authors distinguished three "latent theoretical constructs" related to what they refer to an "ethical prison architecture": humane treatment, autonomy, and stimuli (e.g., prison conditions that are beyond one's control, such as background noise; Engstrom & van Ginneken, 2022). Prison contexts characterized by an "ethical prison architecture," including detention houses, may offer opportunities to secure PHGs (such as agency, life, inner peace, or happiness) and align well with the GLM's core principles; contrary to prisons whose architectural design does not support the well-being of its residents. Given their innovative nature, detention houses in Belgium will be used as a case example.

10.3.1 Detention Houses in Belgium: A Case Example

Detention houses are described by RESCALED (2024) as alternatives for traditional prison settings. RESCALED is a European network organization of 17 countries, that "challenges the concept of 'prison' and proposes the concept of 'detention houses' instead. Detention houses are small-scale, differentiated and community-integrated. Thanks to these three principles, detention houses contribute to sustainable, safe and inclusive societies (RESCALED, 2024, para 1)." Small-scale settings are expected to engender feelings of trust, agency, and taking responsibility. Differentiation refers to support aligned with one's individual needs and aspirations. Community-based means that people stay connected to the communities they belong to.

In Belgium, detention houses were introduced in 2022. In 2024, two detention houses were operational in the cities of Kortrijk and Vorst, with more planned to open in the coming years. Based on the experiences in Kortrijk, the first detention house in Belgium, detention houses are characterized as small-scale centers for people who have been convicted and sentenced to prison for a period of 3 years or less. The residents are assessed as presenting a low safety risk, and persons who have committed sex or terrorist offenses are not eligible (Federal Public Service of Justice [Belgium], 2024). The detained people live together in living groups, aimed at rehabilitating them in society. In a recent presentation at the International Corrections and Prisons Association (ICPA) Annual Conference in Antwerp in 2023, director Petra Colpaert and psychologist Daisy Steen, referred to the following elements that constitute its vision: the contact between staff members and residents (as they are called instead of "prisoners") is based on genuine respect; there is a focus on social skills training; drugs are prohibited, and a drug-free environment is created. The aims and operational functioning of the detention house are based on an integration of the risk-need-responsivity principles (Bonta & Andrews, 2017) and the good lives model. This means that supervision and support of detained people is based on risk assessment and the individual's corresponding level of risk. Besides targeting criminogenic needs/dynamic risk factors and a focus on responsivity (i.e., providing support that is tailored to one's individual needs), equal attention is paid to the resident's PHGs in different domains of life (e.g., education, work, and leisure time) and their prioritized life goals (Colpaert et al., 2023).

Colpaert and Steen (Colpaert et al., 2023) refer to a number of key components of detention house practice guidelines, including dialogue and dynamic safety, autonomy and empowerment, focus on rehabilitation, reducing avoidable pains of imprisonment, and implementation in the local community. These components align well with the core values and principles, knowledge-related assumptions, and intervention and practice guidelines of the GLM as set out by Ward and Durrant (2021) and Willis et al. (2014).

Dialogue and dynamic safety intends to create an environment where people feel safe and secure. This is, for instance, exemplified in being respectful to each other (applicable to residents and staff members), employing a zero-tolerance policy toward aggression, providing a drug-free environment, and small details like addressing someone by their first name instead of their last name or staff not having to wear uniforms as in regular prisons. "Detention counselors," a new role in Belgium, are responsible for the psychosocial support of detained people, while correctional officers are in charge of the procedural safety in correctional facilities. Detention counselors are important in managing the daily living climate where emphasis is on providing the residents with opportunities for autonomy and agency. The function of detention counselors includes providing individual support, facilitating group dynamics and activities, and ensuring a positive living climate. These detention counselors receive specific and comprehensive training about different topics that support individuals (e.g., on mentoring, motivational theories, resilience and coping with stress, suicide prevention); groups (e.g., conflict management); teamwork (e.g., multidisciplinary cooperation); and specific challenges and client profiles (e.g., persons with mental health problems, intellectual disabilities, elderly people, etc). The training also includes a 2-day session on the GLM delivered by and under the supervision of the Belgian members of the international GLM network. The relations between the management, penitentiary staff, psychosocial services, and residents are based on daily communication and mutual respect. This adheres to the GLM core values of human dignity and universal human rights and employs a collaborative approach in developing individual goals. Communication is based on respect and collaboration as is inherent in regular resident meetings, wide and low-threshold accessibility of management and psychosocial service staff, and frequent informal meetings in daily life. Decisions that are important for the residents are explained by the management in the living group, which is less common in regular prisons. Although it cannot be directly assumed that these examples naturally lead to increased agency, these activities may offer opportunities for residents to have a say in how daily life is organized.

Autonomy and empowerment focus on providing residents with opportunities to take active roles in the detention center by working on individual goals included in personalized plans. The purpose is to develop a comprehensive rehabilitation plan (with a legal/judicial objective), that is consistent with practice implications of the GLM, and that aligns with a GLP (i.e., a plan that is directed by the resident). Since the detention house in Kortrijk is still relatively new, the GLM has not yet been fully implemented in developing the rehabilitation plan. Nevertheless, psychologists from the psychosocial service work closely with each resident, and judicial social work services, to create individual plans that encompass all life domains and PHGs. The relatively short stay in a detention center makes it difficult to develop and implement a plan that involves all life domains. Thus, the GLM is currently used as a guiding and inspiring framework for developing a rehabilitation plan, and advice to the judge is based on the RNR and GLM frameworks. The aim is to build understanding among detainees (and other parties involved) about why they committed an offense. Therefore, the rehabilitation plan is created for and with the residents, inspired by the GLM. Much attention is given to what residents consider important and what could help them achieve the PHGs in a prosocial way, rather than focusing solely on risk avoidance, as is often the case in regular prisons. While it may be a big step forward, it is important to keep in mind that the rehabilitation plan differs from a GLP, as the control over a rehabilitation plan lies in the hands of the justice system, not with the resident. For example, if attending an employment-focused course in pursuit of excellence in work becomes a condition included in a rehabilitation plan as part of release requirements, there is a risk it could be perceived by the resident as an obstacle (due to the obligation to attend) rather than as a way to pursue the PHG of excellence in work.

Further, residents take on responsibilities with daily chores (such as cleaning, cooking, and gardening). Residents have more freedom compared to a traditional prison (e.g., they can use cell phones and laptops), and they have keys to their own rooms (Luyten, 2024). Emphasis is placed on individual needs and aspirations, which aligns well with the GLM's core value of human agency. An individual's most valued PHGs are attended to in a collaborative way. For example, residents are involved in managing their financial resources and have opportunities to work outside the facility (Luyten, 2024). The collaborative approach is also exemplified in strong ties and close cooperation with community-based social welfare and vocational services and by mental health treatment and support providers present in the detention facility at scheduled times.

Focus on rehabilitation calls for ongoing emphasis on desirable outcomes in the short, medium, and long terms regarding different aspects of the individual's life (Colpaert & Steen, 2023, in Colpaert et al., 2023) integrated in an individual plan, These different aspects include health, relationships, employment, hobbies and leisure activities, and all other life areas that relate directly to GLM core values (universal human rights); assumptions (providing people with socially accepted means to pursue PHGs); and intervention guidelines (working toward rehabilitation in a collaborative way). The goal of detention house practice is to evolve toward a rehabilitation plan that closely aligns with a GLP where the most important PHGs are included and opportunities are provided to acquire these goods, for example, by referring clients to services that provide specialized care and support. However, a number of challenges must be taken into account: staff in detention houses do not provide therapy themselves (this is offered by external service providers); detention supervisors do not have professional confidentiality and must report what they learn from conversations or observations to the prison management; and many residents have little trust in the justice system due to negative experiences from the past. For this reason, it is important to keep in mind that detention houses also remain a form of confinement, making it doubtful whether a GLP can be fully developed there. However, the stay in a detention house can be seen as an opportunity to develop parts of a plan and, in consultation with the resident, pass this on to specialized care.

Reducing avoidable pains of imprisonment. In his seminal work, Sykes (1958) described what has become widely known as the pains of imprisonment as "the loss of liberty, desirable goods and services, [...] relationships, autonomy, and security" (Shammas, 2017, p. 1). In a detention house, opportunities to avoid and/or reduce these deprivations, are provided. Examples include contact with family, social network, and society at large (e.g., by means of family leave or community work); having a key to one's own room (fostering agency); and taking an active role in the development of a rehabilitation plan (Colpaert & Steen, 2023, in Colpaert et al., 2023). This aligns well with the GLM's ethical values (human dignity, universal human rights, and human agency) and intervention guidelines (working collaboratively).

Implementation in the local community. Detention houses are located in and integrated into local communities, which enables residents to be involved in community activities. Examples include the involvement of residents as volunteers in the city of Kortrijk, community activities such as "Soccer Unites" aimed at bringing together people from within and outside the detention house by means of training together, and guest lectures in neighboring university colleges by residents who testify about their lived experiences. The local embedding also facilitates the organization of community activities that make use of facilities in the detention house for neighborhood-based events or activities where residents can interact with neighbors. For example, the detention house recently hosted a social event with coffee and cake for local residents in the neighborhood. The local placement aligns well with the GLM's core value of universal human rights (e.g., the right of belonging). It also links well with providing opportunities to pursue PHGs in society.

There are clear links between the characteristics of a detention house and the core values and principles, knowledge-related assumptions, and intervention and practice guidelines of the GLM as set out by Ward and Durrant (2021) and Willis et al. (2014). Ward and Durrant (2021) make a distinction between core values and principles, knowledge-related assumptions, and intervention guidelines, and they relate these different levels to the GLM. In terms of core values and principles, the GLM refers to the ethical values of human dignity, universal human rights, and human agency and prudential values corresponding with PHGs and how these are linked with one's well-being. In terms of knowledge-related assumptions, the GLM explores the actions of people to secure PHGs and the obstacles they are confronted with in doing so. In its intervention guidelines, the GLM employs a collaborative approach in developing a GLP (Ward & Durrant, 2021). Willis et al. (2014) developed a coding protocol to assess how well programs comply with the principles of the GLM, based on program aims and orientation, assessment, intervention planning, program content, and program delivery. These domains are summarized in Table 10.1, which aligns detention house practice guidelines with GLM-consistent practices.

Table 10.1 Overview of core values, knowledge-related assumptions and intervention guidelines of GLM-consistent policies. (Adapted from Ward & Durrant, 2021; Willis et al., 2014, p. 74)

Core values and principles		
Ethical values of —human dignity —universal human rights —human agency —well-being enhancement alongside risk reduction		
Knowledge-related assumptions		
Deconstructing dynamic risk factors into agent–action–context impairments, used to infer required internal and external capacities		
Intervention guidelines		
Program domain	*Consistent with GLM*	*Examples detention house Kortrijk*
Program aims and orientation	Focus on dual aim of risk reduction and well-being enhancement; and clear communication about this dual aim	Equal attention is afforded to RNR considerations and the resident's primary goods and prioritized life goals
Assessment	Routine assessment of risk factors	Supervision and support is based on risk assessment and one's corresponding level of risk
	Exploration of future goals and priorities and identification of heavily weighted goods	Comprehensive assessment focuses, from the start, on desirable outcomes in the short, medium, and long terms in regard to different aspects of one's life (Colpaert & Steen, 2023 in Colpaert et al., 2023). These different aspects include health, relationships, employment, hobbies and leisure activities, and all other life areas
	Comprehensive assessment practices canvassing the full range of GLM primary goods	
Intervention planning	Individualized counseling/intervention plans for each client focused on (1) the attainment of heavily weighted goods and (2) the reduction of risk	Criminogenic needs/dynamic risk factors are integrated into the individual plan alongside primary goods and prioritized life goals
Intervention content	Linking modules/activities to attainment of primary goods	Opportunities for contact with family, social network, and society at large (e.g., by means of "family leaves" or community work); having a key of one's own room (fostering agency); and taking an active role in the development of one's personal rehabilitation plan
	Attending to the social ecology and social capital	Detention houses are located and integrated in the local communities, enabling residents to be involved in community activities and facilitating the organization of community activities at the detention house

(continued)

Table 10.1 (continued)

Intervention delivery	Positive counselor characteristics and attitudes	Detention counselors are central to creating a supportive living climate; emphasis is placed on providing residents with opportunities for autonomy and agency
	Collaboration with clients	Residents take an active role in the detention house, including involvement in daily chores (such as cleaning, cooking, and gardening)
	Intervention delivery is individually tailored	Emphasis is placed on individual needs and aspirations, attending to an individual's most valued primary goods in a collaborative way

Implementing the GLM in detention houses requires some vital steps, including training and supervision of staff and maintaining a positive living climate (Colpaert & Steen, 2023 in Colpaert et al., 2023). All staff members (including the detention counselors, directors, and psychologists) of the detention house in Kortrijk participated in a 2-day workshop about the GLM; the psychologists were trained by Tony Ward and Mary Barnao during a 3-day workshop on implementing the GLM; and graduate students of Ghent University Educational Sciences developed materials to follow-up on these trainings (e.g., a video in which the GLM is explained in an accessible way and index cards of the PHGs).[2] Particularly relevant to mention is the work by Yanick Luyten, a graduate student in Special Needs Education and Disability Studies at Ghent University, whose internship program included developing a GLM-based training specifically adapted to the needs of residents in a detention house. The training consists of four sessions, related to the conceptualization of a good life, the primary goods, strengths and obstacles, and the development of a good lives plan (Luyten, 2024). The sessions, that last for about 2.5 h, include information sessions, practical exercises (e.g., by using dice containing the 11 PHGs to elicit interaction on how PHGs can be sought in prosocial ways), interactive group discussions, quizzes (e.g., focused on identifying the appropriate PHG in brief case descriptions), and individual work/self-report registered in a personal work booklet (Luyten, 2024). Although not fully realized yet, the personal booklet is envisioned as a personal document that could support one's rehabilitation process. Further, the GLM is used as a guiding framework to develop a rehabilitation plan mapping one's primary goods by means of observations, self-report, and other activities (e.g., discussion groups with staff members and residents). Bachelor-students in social work (Vives University of Applied Sciences) are involved in supporting these activities (Colpaert et al., 2023).

Although the experiences are generally perceived as positive, Colpaert and Steen (in Colpaert et al., 2023) also identified some challenges related to the further development of detention houses. These include additional training and supervision for detention counselors, further reflection on what can be realistically achieved during (often short) periods of stay, safeguarding continuity of care, and how to address the

---

[2] These materials (in Dutch) are available on request to the authors.

needs of persons with (severe) psychological and/or mental health challenges. It could also be added that detention houses are still a way of confinement governed by the rules of the justice system. This means, for instance, that detention counselors, unlike therapists, are not bound to client confidentiality and that rehabilitation plans in this context differ from fully developed GLPs. Nevertheless, detention houses demonstrate a more humanistic, strengths-based approach to crime that better aligns with the GLM than detaining people in traditional prisons.

10.4 Community-Based Policy Implications

Rehabilitation and reintegration under the auspices of the GLM require an environment that affords opportunities for prosocial attainment of PHGs. When individuals who have offended are identified by communities, opportunities for implementing a good life plan may be compromised (Willis et al., 2010). Indeed, Harris et al. (2019) interviewed 42 men released into the community following convictions for sexual offenses. The GLM was applied retrospectively to interview data to infer the extent to which PHGs were prioritized and pursued. Participants' means to realize primary goods were restricted considerably by their correctional status. Most persons convicted for a crime will complete their sentence and resume the same or similar freedoms they had prior to conviction. Across offense types, notable exceptions include common requirements to disclose convictions when traveling internationally and/or in job applications. However, in the context of sexual offending, contemporary policies can place life-long restrictions on an individual's freedom, their ability to reintegrate, and ultimately their chances to implement a GLP. This section will analyze contemporary community-based policies through a GLM lens.

Residence restrictions and community notification are common contemporary policies that undermine the GLM and, not surprisingly, have failed to reduce rates of sexual reoffending (e.g., Zgoba & Mitchell, 2023). Residence restrictions, enforced in most US states, place restrictions on physical distances an individual can live from areas children commonly congregate in such as schools, day care centers, and parks (Savage & Windsor, 2018). Several studies have documented the adverse impact of residence restrictions on finding housing, seriously undermining the PHG of life. Ultimately, residence restrictions often force individuals with sexual offense convictions to reside in isolated areas away from services and supports, thus impacting their access to sources of multiple primary goods, including relatedness, community, mastery in work, mastery in play, and autonomy (e.g., Levenson, 2008; Levenson & Cotter, 2005).

Community notification similarly reduces individuals' external capacity to realize primary goods. The impetus behind community notification was to increase public safety by providing information about people with convictions for sexual offenses residing in the vicinity. Community notification was based on the premise that providing information would enable neighbors to take proactive steps to protect children and other vulnerable people from victimization (Anderson & Sample, 2008).

Such notification can take varied forms ranging from passive publication that requires community members to search online registers, to active notification whereby authorities directly inform residents that an individual convicted for sexual offending is residing or due to reside in their community. The federal Sex Offender Registration and Notification Act (SORNA) in the USA, commonly known as Megan's law, requires that personal details of "registered sex offenders" (including registrants' photographs and residential addresses) are made publicly accessible via online databases that can be searched by a registrant's name or location. Notification can also take the form of written notifications (e.g., flyers), social media notifications, and community meetings (Cubellis et al., 2018). A recent meta-analysis synthesized results from 18 studies and 474,640 participants to investigate the effects of SORN legislation on adult recidivism over 25 years (Zgoba & Mitchell, 2023). The authors found no significant effects of SORN on sexual or nonsexual recidivism, concluding that SORN legislation had failed to achieve its aim of enhancing community safety. Lasher and McGrath (2012) reviewed eight quantitative studies examining the social and psychological impact of SORN on persons registered across several states ($N = 1503$). Considering social impacts, 44% of registrants reported that they were threatened or harassed by neighbors, 20% reported general threats/harassment, 20% reported job loss, 19% reported loss of housing, 14% reported property damage, and 8% reported physical assaults. Such findings highlight that SORN may compromise desistance processes by obstructing an individual's ability to integrate into a community and implement a GLP. In their critique of SORN legislation, Lussier and Mathesius (2019) commented that "the gap between the empirical literature on sexual offending and the underlying assumptions of American SORN policy cannot be overstated" (p. 111). Indeed, several scholars have contended that from a public perspective, SORN legislation is more symbolic than instrumental (Gesser, 2021; Sample, 2021; Zgoba & Mitchell, 2023).

In many jurisdictions, treatment participation is a requirement of probation or parole. Engaging in rehabilitation programs can certainly support individuals who have offended to strengthen their capacity to access PHGs. Programs can and often do align with the GLM. Moreover, in the context of contemporary policies infringing severely on the prosocial pursuit of PHGs, treatment program attendance can provide a valuable source of goods attainment. Indeed, Harris et al. (2019) found that the primary goods of community and knowledge were commonly attained through group-based sexual offending treatment programs. However, policies requiring individuals to attend a treatment program when they are not actually in need of treatment—including those assessed with a below average risk of reoffending and with sufficiently developed internal capacity to seek out primary goods in adaptive ways—are inconsistent with the GLM (and with RNR principles). In such cases, mandating treatment participation may limit opportunities for prosocial goods attainment through placing restrictions on an individual's availability for employment and other desistance-promoting activities.

Conditions of probation/parole often resemble a list of activities people on probation/parole can't do, who they can't associate with, and where they can't go. Such an avoidant goal focus is entirely inconsistent with the GLM. Among other conditions, many individuals convicted for sexual offenses have a condition prohibiting their viewing of adult pornography, which is a common probation violation in the USA (E. Griffin, personal communication, January 20, 2025). Yet some pornography, and in particular erotica pornography depicting mutually consenting, pleasurable sex with equal power dynamics, might offer an adaptive source of sexual pleasure for clients with no access to sexual partners. Moreover, for clients with limited experience of healthy sexuality, such pornography might offer an educational resource and form part of a therapy plan designed to strengthen internal capacity to seek sexual pleasure in adaptive, prosocial ways (Delmonico & Griffin, 2024).

Generally speaking, policies that help facilitate or provide a direct means of accessing PHGs align well with the GLM. In some jurisdictions, parole/probation conditions prohibit contact between peers with similar offending backgrounds outside of the group treatment setting (e.g., through non-association orders/conditions). Yet elsewhere, there is recognition that such connections can support rehabilitation and reintegration and may be an individual's sole source of the PHG of relatedness. For example, in New Jersey, the Keepsafe program involves individuals transitioning from the state's special treatment unit (STU; established under the New Jersey Sexually Violent Predator Act) to the community to maintain contact with a Keepsafe buddy inside the institution who is vetted and approved by staff to support the released individual. The released individual maintains weekly contact with their Keepsafe buddy, discussing their successes and challenges, and the buddy supports the individual to process difficult situations and implement adaptive coping skills. In addition, the buddy provides regular updates about the individual to the STU, including expressing any concerns they have regarding the individual or their behavior. Any serious concerns are communicated to staff as soon as possible, enabling staff to engage with community-based practitioners and/or parole to intervene or support the individual as necessary. Although not yet formally evaluated, anecdotal evidence suggests that for some individuals, their Keepsafe buddy becomes one of their few friends (Schneider & McBride, 2015).

Also in New Jersey, the STU alumni mentorship program matches STU alumni living in the community with STU residents nearing release. The STU alumni acts as a mentor to the resident as they prepare for discharge, create a discharge plan, and participate in furloughs (temporary releases). The alumni/resident match continues well after the individual has been conditionally discharged into the community, and after 1–2 years the mentee may transition into the role of mentor themselves (Burnett, 2017). Mentors meet with other mentors quarterly as part of a mentor network, which provides a space for mentors to support each other and share resources. Accordingly, the STU alumni mentorship program affords opportunities for accessing several PHGs, including relatedness, community, and knowledge.[3]

---

[3] Circles of Support and Accountability (CoSA; Wilson & Prinzo, 2001) similarly supports acquisition of primary goods through formalized social support networks. Whereas CoSA enlists volunteer support, the New Jersey Keepsafe and Alumni Mentorship programs operate based on peer support.

10.5 Commentary and Conclusion

This chapter has focused on policy implications as they relate to custodial or community sentences, which are typical justice system responses to persons who have offended, and highlighted how correctional policies within institutional and community settings can support or hinder a GLM approach to rehabilitation. By design, most justice system responses restrict to varying degrees an individual's ability to pursue a meaningful, prosocial life. Contemporary responses to crime, therefore, impact on external capacity to attain PHGs for people who have struggled seeking PHGs in prosocial ways throughout their lives. Put another way, they further the distance between people who have offended and mainstream society. If justice system responses were focused instead on offering a pathway for equipping those who have harmed others with the support and resources necessary to live a different life, perhaps their rehabilitation and reintegration would be easier, cheaper, and more effective than what typical justice system responses allow. Comments here are in no way intended to downplay the harm caused by crime, especially violent and sexual offending. Rather, the harm caused by reoffending is what makes investing in systems that steer people away from crime all the more important.

Sentencing options that focus on rehabilitation and (re)integration from the outset offer a better fit with the GLM than retributive approaches to justice that vary by their level of punitiveness and restrictions. For example, justice system responses aligning with principles of therapeutic jurisprudence (Wexler, 2010), which focus on promotion of well-being for all participants in the justice process, are a more natural affiliate with GLM-grounded rehabilitation and reintegration than retributive responses to crime. Examples include restorative justice and problem-solving courts (also referred to as specialist courts), which focus on harm reparation and addressing underlying causes of crime (e.g., through specialist substance abuse or mental health treatment), respectively. At face value, restorative justice may afford opportunities for goods attainment, including agency and inner peace (through bringing together all people impacted by a crime and coming to a decision collaboratively about appropriate reparations), whereas problem-solving courts may provide opportunities for strengthening internal capacity to attain primary goods in prosocial ways. Research on these alternative approaches to justice is limited, in part due to an absence—until recently—of a sound theoretical framework outlining what constitutes therapeutic jurisprudence in action (Howieson, 2023).

10.5.1 Conclusion

This chapter has offered specific examples of GLM-consistent (and inconsistent) correctional policies. Many contemporary correctional policies reflect reactive responses to high profile, low base rate crimes as reflected in their naming (e.g., "Megan's law" in the USA, "Sarah's law in the UK). Unlike international government responses to the Covid-19 pandemic, they are not empirically informed, or effective in preventing crime. Encouragingly however, as highlighted throughout this chapter, some jurisdictions have enacted promising policies that better align with the GLM but remain in need of empirical research to ascertain their effectiveness.

GLM-consistent policies comply with the core values and principles, knowledge-related assumptions, and intervention guidelines of the GLM as set out by Ward and Durrant (2021) and Willis et al. (2014). The core values and principles relate to the ethical values of human dignity, universal human rights, human agency, and well-being enhancement alongside risk reduction. The knowledge-related assumptions refer to deconstructing DRFs into agent–action–context impairments used to infer required internal and external capacities. As for intervention guidelines, the GLM employs a collaborative approach in developing a GLP and supporting its execution (Ward & Durrant, 2021).

Blanket, one-size-fits-all policies that dictate what people can't do, where they can't go, and who they can't associate with undermine a GLM approach to correctional rehabilitation. Although it may be justified (at least pragmatically) to prohibit someone with a long history of offending against stranger children to live nearby a primary school, the same policy is not relevant for someone who offended against a family member, or for a man in his late teens who was convicted for statutory rape against a former 15-year-old girlfriend. Similarly, it would be contraindicated for someone who has struggled with alcohol addiction to live next door to a liquor store. Through the lens of the GLM, it becomes apparent that highly restrictive policies may unnecessarily hinder the pursuit of primary goods in such a way that they halt effective (re)integration into society and potentially reinforce an offender identity. Without meaningful, adaptive means through which to secure primary goods, there is the very real possibility that individuals will return to previous ways of living. The GLM calls for flexibility in the application of crime management policies, with consideration extending beyond what someone must avoid to how they can be supported to live a better life than that they have known.

References

Ackerman, A. R., Harris, A. J., Levenson, J. S., & Zgoba, K. (2011). Who are the people in your neighborhood? A descriptive analysis of individuals on public sex offender registries. *International Journal of Law and Psychiatry, 34*(3), 149–159. https://doi.org/10.1016/j.ijlp.2011.04.001

Anderson, A. L., & Sample, L. L. (2008). Public awareness and action resulting from sex offender community notification laws. *Criminal Justice Policy Review, 19*(4), 371–396. https://doi.org/10.1177/0887403408316705

B4U-ACT. (2019). *Learn: Know the facts*. B4U-ACT. https://www.b4uact.org/know-the-facts/

Bonta, J., & Andrews, D. A. (2017). *The psychology of criminal conduct* (6th ed.). Routledge.

Burnett, H. (2017). *STU Alumni Mentorship Program: Program description*.

Cheliotis, L. K. (2008). Reconsidering the effectiveness of temporary release: A systematic review. *Aggression and Violent Behavior, 13*(3), 153–168. https://doi.org/10.1016/j.avb.2008.02.004

Chiricos, T. E. D., Barrick, K., Bales, W., & Bontrager, S. (2007). The labeling of convicted felons and its consequences for recidivism. *Criminology, 45*, 547–581. https://doi.org/10.1111/j.1745-9125.2007.00089.x
Chisadza, C., Clance, M., & Gupta, R. (2021). Government effectiveness and the COVID-19 pandemic. *Sustainability, 13*(6), 3042. https://www.mdpi.com/2071-1050/13/6/3042
Colpaert, P., Steen, D., & Vandevelde, S. (2023). Workshop on the Good Lives Model. Workshop presented at the Annual International Corrections & Prisons Associations (ICPA) Conference, 22–27 October 2023, Antwerp, Belgium. Accessed July 2024, from https://icpa.org/resource/the-implementation-of-good-lives-model-in-daily-life-and-rehabilitation-of-offenders.html
Cubellis, M. A., Walfield, S. M., & Harris, A. J. (2018). Collateral consequences and effectiveness of sex offender registration and notification: Law enforcement perspectives. *International Journal of Offender Therapy and Comparative Criminology, 62*(4), 1080–1106. https://doi.org/10.1177/0306624x16667574
Delmonico, D., & Griffin, E. (2024). #illegalimages: Treating individuals who view child sexual abuse media. In *Association for the Treatment and Prevention of Sexual Abuse (ATSA) Annual Conference*.
Dunn, D. S., & Andrews, E. E. (2015). Person-first and identity-first language: Developing psychologists' cultural competence using disability language. *American Psychologist, 70*, 255–264. https://doi.org/10.1037/a0038636
Engstrom, K. V., & van Ginneken, E. F. J. C. (2022). Ethical prison architecture: A systematic literature review of prison design features related to wellbeing. *Space and Culture, 25*(3), 479–503. https://doi.org/10.1177/12063312221104211
Federal Public Service of Justice (Belgium). (2024). *Detentiehuizen*. https://justitie.belgium.be/nl/themas/gevangenissen/belgische_gevangenissen/detentiehuizen
Gesser, N. (2021). What you expect is not what you get: The antitherapeutic impact of sex offender community notification meetings on community members. *Psychology, Public Policy, & Law, 27*, 432–447. https://doi.org/10.1037/law0000303
Harris, D. A., Pedneault, A., & Willis, G. M. (2019). The pursuit of primary human goods in men desisting from sexual offending. *Sexual Abuse, 31*, 197–219. https://doi.org/10.1177/1079063217729155
Howieson, J. A. (2023). A framework for the evidence-based practice of therapeutic jurisprudence: A legal therapeutic alliance. *International Journal of Law and Psychiatry, 89*, 101906. https://doi.org/10.1016/j.ijlp.2023.101906
Jewkes, Y. (2018). Just design: Healthy prisons and the architecture of hope. *Australian & New Zealand Journal of Criminology, 51*(3), 319–338. https://doi.org/10.1177/0004865818766768
Lasher, M. P., & McGrath, R. J. (2012). The impact of community notification on sex offender reintegration: A quantitative review of the research literature. *International Journal of Offender Therapy and Comparative Criminology, 56*(1), 6–28. https://doi.org/10.1177/0306624x10387524
Levenson, J. S. (2008). Collateral consequences of sex offender residence restrictions. *Criminal Justice Studies, 21*, 153–166. https://doi.org/10.1080/14786010802159822
Levenson, J. S., & Cotter, L. P. (2005). The impact of sex offender residence restrictions: 1,000 feet from danger or one step from absurd? *International Journal of Offender Therapy and Comparative Criminology, 49*, 168–178. https://doi.org/10.1177/0306624X04271304
Luigi, M., Dellazizzo, L., Giguère, C.-É., Goulet, M.-H., & Dumais, A. (2020). Shedding light on "the Hole": A systematic review and meta-analysis on adverse psychological effects and mortality following solitary confinement in correctional settings [Systematic Review]. *Frontiers in Psychiatry, 11*. https://doi.org/10.3389/fpsyt.2020.00840
Luigi, M., Dellazizzo, L., Giguère, C., Goulet, M. H., Potvin, S., & Dumais, A. (2022). Solitary confinement of inmates associated with relapse into any recidivism including violent crime: A systematic review and meta-analysis. *Trauma, Violence, & Abuse, 23*(2), 444–456. https://doi.org/10.1177/1524838020957983

Lussier, P., & Mathesius, J. (2019). Trojan horse policies: Sexual predators, SORN laws and the American experience. *Psychology, Crime & Law, 25*(2), 133–156. https://doi.org/10.1080/1068316X.2018.1503666
Luyten, Y. (2024). *Personal Communication: Presentation about the detention house in Kortrijk.* Unpublished course material.
Mathlin, G., Freestone, M., & Jones, H. (2024). Factors associated with successful reintegration for male offenders: A systematic narrative review with implicit causal model. *Journal of Experimental Criminology, 20*(2), 541–580. https://doi.org/10.1007/s11292-022-09547-5
RESCALED. (2024). *RESCALED – European movement for detention houses*. Retrieved July 2024, from https://www.rescaled.org/
Restivo, E., & Lanier, M. M. (2015). Measuring the contextual effects and mitigating factors of labeling theory. *Justice Quarterly, 32*, 116–141. https://doi.org/10.1080/07418825.2012.756115
Sample, L. L. (2021). The public and SORN Laws. In J. J. Prescott & W. Logan (Eds.), *Sex offender registration and community notification laws: An empirical evaluation* (pp. 59–77). Cambridge University Press. https://doi.org/10.1017/9781108328425.006
Savage, J., & Windsor, C. (2018). Sex offender residence restrictions and sex crimes against children: A comprehensive review. *Aggression and Violent Behavior, 43*, 13–25. https://doi.org/10.1016/j.avb.2018.08.002
Schneider, J. E., & McBride, J. (2015). *The role of support networks in "Keeping Safe" in the community*. Association for the Treatment and Prevention of Sexual Abuse (ATSA) Annual Conference, Montreal, Canada.
Shammas, V. L. (2017). Pains of imprisonment. In *The encyclopedia of corrections* (pp. 1–5). https://doi.org/10.1002/9781118845387.wbeoc020
Silverthorn, R., & Zgoba, K. M. (2024). Unlocking the truth: Exploring the impacts of solitary confinement on recidivism and the need for mental health support for individuals with mental illnesses. *American Journal of Criminal Justice*. Advance online publication. https://doi.org/10.1007/s12103-024-09771-x
Sykes, G. (1958). *The society of captives: A study of a maximum security prison*. Princeton University Press.
Ward, T., & Birgden, A. (2007). Human rights and correctional clinical practice. *Aggression and Violent Behavior, 12*(6), 628–643. https://doi.org/10.1016/j.avb.2007.05.001
Ward, T., & Durrant, R. (2021). Practice frameworks in correctional psychology: Translating causal theories and normative assumptions into practice. *Aggression and Violent Behavior, 58*, 101612. https://doi.org/10.1016/j.avb.2021.101612
Ward, T., & Salmon, K. (2009). The ethics of punishment: Correctional practice implications. *Aggression and Violent Behavior, 13*, 239–247. https://doi.org/10.1016/j.avb.2009.03.009
Wexler, D. B. (2010). Therapeutic jurisprudence and its application to criminal justice research and development. *Irish Probation Journal, 7*, 94.
Willis, G. M. (2018). Why call someone by what we don't want them to be? The ethics of labelling in forensic/correctional psychology. *Psychology, Crime & Law, 24*, 727–743. https://doi.org/10.1080/1068316X.2017.1421640
Willis, G. M., Levenson, J. S., & Ward, T. (2010). Desistance and attitudes towards sex offenders: Facilitation or hindrance? *Journal of Family Violence, 25*, 545–556. https://doi.org/10.1007/s10896-010-9314-8
Willis, G. M., Ward, T., & Levenson, J. S. (2014). The Good Lives Model (GLM): An evaluation of GLM operationalization in North American treatment programs. *Sexual Abuse, 26*, 58–81. https://doi.org/10.1177/1079063213478202
Wilson, R. J., & Prinzo, M. (2001). Circles of support: A restorative justice initiative. *Journal of Psychology & Human Sexuality, 13*(3–4), 59–77. https://doi.org/10.1300/J056v13n03_05
Zgoba, K. M., & Mitchell, M. M. (2023). The effectiveness of Sex Offender Registration and Notification: A meta-analysis of 25 years of findings. *Journal of Experimental Criminology, 19*, 71–96. https://doi.org/10.1007/s11292-021-09480-z

Chapter 11
Conclusions

This book is intended to be a one-stop resource for clinicians wanting to develop a working understanding of the good lives model (GLM) and its core values, knowledge assumptions, and practice guidelines. It represents the definitive version of the model to date, and we have tried to integrate the numerous theoretical and practice innovations that have appeared since the model's first appearance over 20 years ago. The GLM is a practice framework developed within the science-informed intervention tradition and underpinned by the foundational values of human dignity and human rights.

The key take-home points of this book are as follows. First, forensic and correctional clients are, in many respects, indistinguishable from the practitioners who work with them in that they are people like us. They have the same set of basic needs, aspirations, and desire to be treated with respect and to have a chance of achieving the things that matter most to them. Second, clinicians should consider that people within the criminal justice system who participate in intervention programs want the possibility of better lives beyond the promise of less harmful ones. It is not just about targeting risk factors and learning to comply with laws and social norms. Clients have every right to ask: What will I get out of therapy? How will the long and personally confronting process of change benefit me? We should be able to give positive and constructive answers to these questions. Third, strengths-based programs, such as those derived from the GLM, can help people live meaningfully, alongside reducing their risk of harming others. This approach works by basing intervention plans on clients' core values and associated practical identities and by providing them with the internal and external resources to achieve what they value most in the world. Fourth, the model of human nature underlying GLM practice is that of culturally saturated, physically embodied, relational, and extended agency. Individuals actively shape their environments which, in turn, shape them. Clinicians need to take this into account in every aspect of their work and realize that during the intervention process they become an integral part of clients' extended cognitive and affective systems. Fifth, a strong client–therapist relationship is a pivotal and

T. Ward et al., *The Good Lives Model of Correctional Rehabilitation*,
Advances in Preventing and Treating Violence and Aggression,
https://doi.org/10.1007/978-3-031-95559-4_11

crucial precondition of enduring change. Certainly, practitioners need to master a wide range of technical skills to be effective in what they do; however, without a good alliance, therapy is likely to be ineffective. Therapy is not an algorithmic process. Instead, it is fundamentally a human relationship in which clients reveal what kind of shape they would like their lives to take, while therapists help to design and construct the resulting "building." That is, clinicians help their clients find a viable way of living well within the constraints of human obligations and entitlements. As practitioners, we do not see ourselves as normative police officers who exercise authorities over people's lives; rather, we look at clients as fellow travelers who are all unique subjects with their own prioritized goals. Finally, the GLM is an ecological model and reminds practitioners and policymakers that effective intervention plans should consider the social, physical, and cultural ecosystems clients are likely to be living in once they leave prison or complete their programs. The ecosystems of services (e.g., prisons, forensic hospitals) impact on the effectiveness of clients' intervention plans, particularly when they are detained for lengthy periods of time. Ultimately, services should align their processes and practices, as much as is realistically possible, to support the core values and principles of the GLM, including a focus on human rights. There is little point in delivering state-of-the-art intervention programs and then releasing individuals into hostile, unforgiving, and rejecting communities. In this context, society and its policymakers are responsible for creating opportunities for all people to be able to implement their GLP in a prosocial way.

Much of what therapists do is aspirational, and they often battle against the odds when working with clients within the criminal justice system. All we can do is remind ourselves of the above key points and work locally to effect change in clients' lives and within the wider systems in which we work. Clinicians should resist the temptation of demonizing individuals who commit crimes. They must be aware that they can use their position and the use of psychology oppressively (and should not practice it in this way) and be open to the possibility that with our help these individuals can turn their lives around. Such openness requires a willingness to acknowledge the possibility of clients' past trauma and social disadvantage while accepting that ultimately, they must take responsibility for working on their problems. It all comes down to the twin components of human rights which form the ethical center of the GLM: entitlements to psychological, physical, and social resources along with the obligations to consider the core interests of other people when deciding how to act. The two components of human rights align remarkably well with the GLM's twin goals of client well-being enhancement and risk reduction.

It is our hope that this book will give practitioners some of the tools they need to offer services constructively in ways that reflect these foundational values when working with individuals who have committed crimes. We also hope that it may inspire legislators to develop and implement rehabilitation policies that support people who have offended to pursue primary goods in prosocial and personally fulfilling ways. As indicated above, GLM-inspired crime management policies focus on providing opportunities that enable people to build a good life, rather than merely ensuring the avoidance of criminal behavior.

We offer a challenge to readers to help build and transform practice and policies for the better in the years ahead, such that good lives are attainable to all. We invite you to join us in this quest, following in the footsteps of Bill Marshall, to whom we have dedicated this book.

Appendices

Appendix A: Exploratory Interview Questions

1. Tell me a bit about yourself and your life just before you came into hospital/service. (e.g., what were you doing before you came into hospital/service? What did you enjoy doing? Who did you spend your time with? What was important to you?)
2. When you were young, what did you dream about becoming later in life? What were the goals that you had for yourself? What did you do to meet those goals? Were some goals more important to you than others? Which ones were and why? What got in the way of meeting your goals?
3. Who are the people who have had the most influence on your life? Why?
4. If you could be anyone at all (e.g., people you know, famous or infamous people, fictional characters), who would you most want to be like? Why? Who would you least want to be like? Why?
5. What sort of life would you like for yourself in the future? What would you like to achieve? What have you always wanted to achieve?
6. If you could wake up one day and things were just as you wanted them to be, what would it be like? Where would you be? What would you be doing? How would you be feeling? Who would you be with? What things wouldn't you be doing?

T. Ward et al., *The Good Lives Model of Correctional Rehabilitation*, Advances in Preventing and Treating Violence and Aggression,
https://doi.org/10.1007/978-3-031-95559-4

Appendix B: Assessment of Primary Goods

Life physical well-being: Being healthy and meeting basic needs

What did the person do to be healthy and meet basic needs? (*means*) e.g., attending to diet, exercise, sleep, taking medication, criminal activity, looking out for threats to well-being or safety	Importance of being healthy and meeting basic needs (*Importance*)	How effective were the things the person did to be healthy and meet basic needs? (*Relationship to offending/mental illness*)	What does this tell us about the person? (*Internal and external strengths and obstacles*)
		What worked well?	Internal strengths
			External strengths
	High	What didn't work well?	Internal obstacles
	Moderate		External obstacles
	Low		
		What activities/ behaviors (i.e., means) created problems for the person or others? What problems? Were these activities/ behaviors related to mental illness/ offending?	

Relationships: Connections to others through relationships with family, friends, romantic partners, and others

What did the person do to have relationships and friendships? (*means*) e.g., spend time with their family, drink or play sport with their mates, have an intimate/ sexual relationship, support other people, be a member of a gang	Importance of having relationships (*Importance*)	How effective were the things the person did to have relationships and friendships? (*Relationship to offending/mental illness*)	What does this tell us about the person? (*Internal and external strengths and obstacles*)
		What worked well?	Internal strengths
			External strengths
	High	What didn't work well?	Internal obstacles
	Moderate		External obstacles
	Low	What activities/behaviors (i.e., means) created problems for the person or others? What problems? Were these activities/ behaviors related to mental illness/offending?	

Community: Belonging to social groups or groups with shared interests

What did the person do to be part of a group? (*means*) e.g., go to church, join a gang, belong to a sports team, contribute to their community	Importance of being part of a group (*Importance*)	How effective were the things the person did to be part of a group? (*Relationship to offending/mental illness*)	What does this tell us about the person? (*Internal and external strengths and obstacles*)
		What worked well?	Internal strengths
			External strengths
		What didn't work well?	Internal obstacles
	High		External obstacles
	Moderate		
	Low		
		What activities/behaviors (i.e., means) created problems for the person or others? What problems? Were these activities/behaviors related to mental illness/offending?	

Mastery in Work

What did the person do to be good at work? (*means*) e.g., get education or training to become better at a job; do voluntary work to pick up work skills	Importance of being good at work (*Importance*)	How effective were the things the person did to be good at work? (*Relationship to offending/mental illness*)	What does this tell us about the person? (*Internal and external strengths and obstacles*)
		What worked well?	Internal strengths
			External strengths
		What didn't work well?	Internal obstacles
	High		External obstacles
	Moderate		
	Low		
		What activities/behaviors (i.e., means) created problems for the person or others? What problems? Were these activities/behaviors related to mental illness/offending?	

Mastery in Play: Being good at and enjoying leisure or recreational activities

What did the person do for recreation/leisure? (*means*) e.g., play sports, do hobbies, brew their own beer, get stoned with mates	Importance of recreation/ leisure (*Importance*)	How effective were the things the person did for recreation/ leisure work? (*Relationship to offending/mental illness*)	What does this tell us about the person? (*Internal and external strengths and obstacles*)
		What worked well?	Internal strengths
			External strengths
	High	What didn't work well?	Internal obstacles
	Moderate		External obstacles
	Low		
		What activities/behaviors (e.g., means) created problems for the person or others? What problems? Were these activities/behaviors related to mental illness/offending?	

Creativity: The desire to have novelty or innovation in one's life

What did the person do to be creative? (*means*) e.g., trying new things that they have not done before, artistic activities, creating a product, experimenting with new drugs	Importance of being creative (*Importance*)	How effective were the things the person did to be creative? (*Relationship to offending/mental illness*)	What does this tell us about the person? (*Internal and external strengths and obstacles*)
		What worked well?	Internal strengths
			External strengths
	High	What didn't work well?	Internal obstacles
	Moderate		External obstacles
	Low		
		What activities/behaviors (i.e., means) created problems for the person or others? What problems? Were these activities/ behaviors related to mental illness/offending?	

Agency: Directing one's own life

What did the person do to have personal choice or be independent? (*means*) e.g., be assertive, break rules, control others, work on a goal, feel that they have to get others before they get you	Importance of being independent or having personal choice (*Importance*)	How effective were the things the person did to be independent and have personal choice? (*Relationship to offending/mental illness*)	What does this tell us about the person? (*Internal and external strengths and obstacles*)
		What worked well?	Internal strengths
			External strengths
	High	What didn't work well?	Internal obstacles
	Moderate		External obstacles
	Low	What activities/ behaviors (i.e., means) created problems for the person or others? What problems? Were these activities/ behaviors related to mental illness/ offending?	

Knowledge: Desire for information and understanding about oneself and the world

What did the person do to get knowledge or information and find out things? (*means*) e.g., placing importance on education/personally relevant information, learning about themselves in therapy, reading the newspaper	Importance of knowing things and being informed (*Importance*)	How effective were the things the person did to get knowledge or information? (*Relationship to offending/ mental illness*)	What does this tell us about the person? (*Internal and external strengths and obstacles*)
		What worked well?	Internal strengths
			External strengths
	High	What didn't work well?	Internal obstacles
	Moderate		External obstacles
	Low		
		What activities/behaviors (i.e., means) created problems for the person or others? What problems? Were these activities/ behaviors related to mental illness/offending?	

Inner Peace: Feeling calm and relaxed and trying to reduce stress

What did the person do to feel calm and relaxed? (*means*) e.g., listen to music, talk to others, exercise, use drugs, alcohol, or medication, hurt themselves, shut down	Importance of being calm and relaxed (*Importance*)	How effective were the things the person did to feel calm and relaxed? (*Relationship to offending/ mental illness*)	What does this tell us about the person? (*Internal and external strengths and obstacles*)
		What worked well?	Internal strengths
			External strengths
	High	What didn't work well?	Internal obstacles
	Moderate		External obstacles
	Low		
		What activities/behaviors (i.e., means) created problems for the person or others? What problems? Were these activities/ behaviors related to mental illness/offending?	

States of happiness and pleasure: Feeling content or experiencing pleasure

What did the person do to feel happy? (*means*) e.g., listen to music, use drugs or alcohol, have sex, eat, shop	Importance of feeling happy (*Importance*)	How effective were the things the person did to feel happy? (*Relationship to offending/ mental illness*)	What does this tell us about the person? (*Internal and external strengths and obstacles*)
		What worked well?	Internal strengths
			External strengths
	High	What didn't work well?	Internal obstacles
	Moderate		External obstacles
	Low		
		What activities/behaviors (i.e., means) created problems for the person or others? What problems? Were these activities/ behaviors related to mental illness/offending?	

Spirituality: Finding meaning or a purpose in life

What did the person do to get a sense of meaning in life? (*means*) e.g., being a parent, taking part in religious activities, reading or studying spiritual materials, meditating, praying or studying spiritual materials	Importance of having a sense of meaning in life (*Importance*)	How effective were the things the person did to get meaning in life? (*Relationship to offending/ mental illness*)	What does this tell us about the person? (*Internal and external strengths and obstacles*)
		What worked well?	Internal strengths
			External strengths
	High	What didn't work well?	Internal obstacles
	Moderate		External obstacles
	Low		
		What activities/behaviors (i.e., means) created problems for the person or others? What problems? Were these activities/ behaviors related to mental illness/offending?	

Appendix C: GLM Mapping Table

Primary Goods	**Importance (high, moderate, low)**	**Internal Strengths**	**Internal obstacles**	**External Strengths**	**External Obstacles**	**Means (adaptive and maladaptive)**	**Relationship to offending/ mental illness (related, unrelated, protective)**
Life							
Relatedness							
Community							
Mastery in Work							
Mastery in Play							
Creativity							
Agency							
Knowledge							
Inner Peace							
States of Happiness & Pleasure							
Spirituality							

Appendix D: Rehabilitation Plan

Primary goods *Indicate priorities	**Interventions**		
	Short term: 3 months	Medium term: 6 months	Long term: 1 year or more
Life			
Relatedness			
Community			
Mastery in work			
Mastery in play			
Creativity			
Agency			
Knowledge			
Inner Peace			
States of Happiness and Pleasure			
Spirituality			

Appendix E: Glossary of Good Lives Model Terms

Coherence. There are two types of coherence problems that can occur in a person's Good Life Plan: *horizontal coherence* and *vertical coherence*. Horizontal coherence refers to the extent to which goods are explicitly related to each other in a mutually consistent and enabling way. Vertical coherence means that PHGs require hierarchical clarity or ranking in terms of priority and importance. The GLM does not specify the level of importance assigned to each PHG. This is an entirely individual process, informed by each person's preferences, skills, likes and dislikes, social norms, and cultural values.

Good Life goals (GLGs) future-oriented secondary goods. Whereas primary human goods can take the form of actions, states, experiences, or ways of being, GLGs are the more concrete plans for achieving the goods. In forming an intervention plan, GLGs can be established in ways that are specific, measurable, achievable, relevant, and time-bound. It is not uncommon for specific Good Life goals to map onto (i.e., provide a source of) multiple PHGs, and organizing the intervention plan around Good Life goals can therefore support generation of an individualized and coherent intervention plan.

Good Life Plan (GLP). A GLP is a coherent set of strategies for achieving a good life. GLPs can be implicit (that is, beyond the awareness of the individual) or explicit (such as those developed in therapy). Examples of GLPs can be found in Chap. 8.

Obstacles. The GLM defines four kinds of obstacles: problematic *means,* where the instrumental or secondary goods used in pursuit of PHGs are maladaptive and/or harmful; narrow *scope*, where an individual focuses narrowly on selected PHG(s) and neglects other prioritized goods; *conflict* or a lack of coherence in means used to attain different PHGs, or in the prioritization of PHGs; and finally, problems with *capacity* within the client (internal capacity) and/or in their environment (external capacity) to seek out primary goods in adaptive, meaningful ways.

Practical identity. This a description of oneself in which individuals find value in aspects of themselves and their lives. Examples include being a university professor in the service of the PHG of knowledge or as a car mechanic where the core value is that of mastery at work. What is particularly pertinent for therapists is that if a person is unable to find ways of achieving their most highly weighted PHG, they are likely to feel their lives lack meaning.

Primary human goods (PHGs). These are outcomes that individuals seek for their own sake (and that have intrinsic value) and in personally meaningful ways. Within the GLM, all human actions are directly or indirectly linked to the seeking of PHGs, including criminal and anti-social behavior. The goals individuals set for themselves are therefore targeted toward the securing of a human good or goods within the contexts in which they live.

Secondary human goods (means). Individuals specific ways of seeking and achieving primary goods in their day-to-day lives; strategies and concrete behaviors associated with a particular good such as seeking the PHG of intimacy by having sex with a child or a sense of autonomy though the physical and psychological domination of another person.

Appendix F: Optimizing GLM Language for Different Settings

Practitioners sometimes experience the language of the PHGs as too broad for use as therapy goals. Various attempts to adjust the language accordingly have taken place over the years. The following have emerged in practice over the years, with some having been mentioned in Yates and Prescott (2011) and are offered below.

- Life => Life: living and surviving
- Knowledge => Knowledge: learning and knowing
- Mastery in play => Mastery in play
- Mastery in work => Mastery in work
- Agency => Autonomy and/or independence
- Inner peace => Inner peace or peace of mind
- Relatedness => Relationships and friendships
- Community => Being part of a community
- Spirituality => Spirituality or having meaning and purpose
- States of happiness and pleasure => Happiness and pleasure
- Creativity => Creativity

References

Yates, P. M., & Prescott, D. S. (2011). *Preventing sexual re-offending: A workbook for building a better life*. Brandon, VT: Safer Society Press.

Index

T. Ward et al., *The Good Lives Model of Correctional Rehabilitation*, Advances in Preventing and Treating Violence and Aggression,
https://doi.org/10.1007/978-3-031-95559-4

The manufacturer's authorised representative in the EU is Springer Nature Customer Service Centre GmbH, Europaplatz 3, 69115 Heidelberg, Germany. If you have any concerns regarding our products, please contact ProductSafety@springernature.com

Printed and bound by CPI Group (UK) Ltd, Croydon, CR0 4YY
01/10/2026
02225971-0004